Between
Life & Death

Surviving the Darkness

Dale M. Bayliss

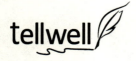

Tellwell Talent
www.tellwell.ca

ISBN
978-1-77370-313-8 (Hardcover)
978-1-77370-312-1 (Paperback)
978-1-77370-314-5 (eBook)

Dedicated to my EMS Family and Friends

"Between Life & Death" is dedicated to the amazing people that I've had the privilege to work with throughout my long career; you are all very precious to me and you all make my life complete. Thank you for helping to make the world just a little better off; you all matter.

EMS Members

EMS Dispatchers

Hospital Staff

STARS Crews and Pilots

Rotary and Fixed Wing Personal

Volunteer / Paid Firefighters

The Good Samaritans

Parks Canada

Search and Rescue

Armed Forces

RCMP

Sheriffs, Police, and Peace Officers

Volunteer Rescue Groups

The Dedicated Community

EMS Boards

All EMS Volunteers

Thank You My Friend

Between Life and Death "Book Two" was completely funded for publication by Rob Hastie who is a lifelong friend and one of my many past paramedic students. Rob could see my dream and was one of the few that made this book come to life. I will always be in your debt, my friend.

The help from our friends keeps us heading in the right direction as we live life. There is not one of us that can survive the chaos that life creates without a partner and from peer support. No matter what we faced we faced it together. That is what mattered.

"Sometimes we need to bend the rules to save a life, but we should not break our moral code, destroy our ethics, or lose our soul along the way."

Dale M. Bayliss

Table of Contents

Prelude

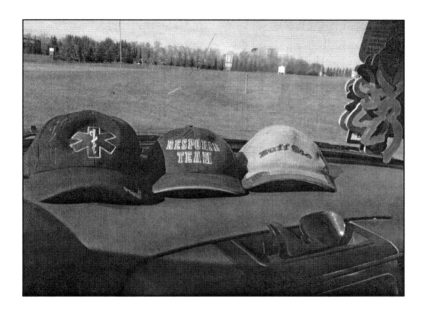

One of the main reasons for writing this book was to ultimately save one of my fellow EMS members from harm's way. We need to work together to be able to help all of us through some very troubling times when needed. My biggest wish was to help my EMS family members be able to face the repeated stressful challenges with a better built in coping mechanism. We also need to build a backup system that we have ready to help us on our worst day. Everyone needs a backup plan. Sadly, we have lost many of our EMS family members around the world over the years because we had no idea what Post Traumatic Stress Disorder (PTSD) or Compassion

Fatigue was or how we should deal with it after the tragic events have occurred. We are just recently realizing the impact of the effects of trauma, disasters, pain and repeated exposure to stressful events on all EMS, Police, Firefighters and Military staff. Nothing is more important than us trying to protect our fellow co-workers from personal or intentional self-harm.

We will all need to work very hard physically, emotionally and mentally all while we respond to the many horrific and complex calls. We often will need to break our endurance limits to simply help or to save many lives. "We need to work as a team to change destiny just as we need to do what's right for our patients despite the protocols in place! Patients are much more complex than any one protocol. In the end, it's the teamwork at a Basic Life Support (BLS) and with the Advanced Life Support (ALS) level that makes the Emergency Medical Services (EMS) team work better to help people in need of medical care."

This book is partly fictional but is based from many real-life stories from my past career in the Emergency Medical Services (EMS), but also as a Flight Paramedic / Flight Nurse and from my many years responding in the Fire Services as a volunteer firefighter. It's a strong inspirational, educational as well as an honest dedication to the people who help others in need 24/7 – 365 days-a-year with no personal reservations. We do what we can so others may live.

Many EMS members would not or can't do this job for just the money, for that would not ever be enough. We do it to help others for it is our own personal calling in life. In many cases, we are all that keeps people away from an untimely death. We maintain life whenever possible at all cost. We are the ones that stand by your side, we fight your personal battles to defeat illness and we try to sustain life as long as possible outside of the hospital settings in almost all cases.

You need to know we all are entitled to fall apart or to feel pain. You need to know and then understand that after responding to some of the most horrific calls in your career it's okay to feel bad. It's also okay to feel hurt or to lose faith in our world after a very bad day. We all have the potential to be emotionally affected and can also be physically broken from time to time from repeatedly seeing severe pain, traumatic injuries, fatal injuries and death. That is the price we must pay for helping the people in need from time to time. That being said please never give up your hope for the one person out there that needs you the most. After all that is the reason we do what we do for others. We need to be able to help each other from time to time when we get knocked down by life's personal tragic, horrific or unexpected events.

My second goal is that I want everyone in EMS to work more as a team at all levels of care. We simply need each other to do our job well. We need each other to help us throughout the good and bad calls to do our ultimate best. I would also like to provide some self-help wisdom to increase your coping skills while facing the repeated daily disasters we will see 24/7 which is (twenty-four hours a day as well as seven days a week). When we respond as a team we can increase our strength and endurance to handle the hard calls.

When we work together we add an extra level of protection for each other before, during or after the calls. Nothing we do in EMS is a solo experience for this industry is a made up of unique special teams to ensure our profession exceeds the minimum standards, thus our patients and our communities receive the optimal level of care. In my mind, the BLS and the ALS practitioners should also be an equal part of every team. It needs to be just be one team. My ultimate inner hope is to bring our EMS world and our practitioners just a little bit closer together as a group all while getting the public on our side.

I will introduce all non-medical personnel to a very realistic EMS perspective that displays the level of difficulties we face from day to day on some of our scariest or difficult calls. I will then show you the level of complexity within our job and then I will show you the real dedication needed by our members to help the people in need.

Somehow, I want to show the world that with a team approach we can be more effective as a profession. We need to be just one big family, a team of one. It should simply be a golden rule. The first golden rule in EMS should be: *"All for one and one for all."* In everything we do. We need to stand and show the world we are one unified group and that our profession is worthy of receiving the mutual respect from our fellow allied health care workers. We require their ongoing support in order for us to continually provide the highest standard of care in the world.

We can't stand and fight this battle alone and we can't make our profession grow unless we evolve into an improved dynamic EMS system along with our constantly changing complex health care world. We need to spread our profession towards community care, while also increasing our educational standards and by evolving into our solo entity as Emergency Medical Specialist.

Together we must face the many medical or traumatic disasters and make the best of any every situation. This book will let you walk my 2300 km walk during my year all while trying to be better than I used to be. Many of my co-workers and my significant friends can see my true determination to change the world. I want them all on my side and we as a team can change the world one person at a time.

This book will share my belief that with time, extra effort and pure determination we'll change the EMS world to be the best it can be as we face the many challenges of a broken world together as a solo team. Just maybe we can prevent some of the ongoing global disasters by increasing our involvement in public education, increased public awareness campaigns and by working with our communities at a professional but an intimate level to prevent the future misadventures heading our way. We can't keep providing reactionary medicine as we have in the past, we need to work towards the prevention of illness and injuries at all cost.

Along our career pathways my fellow Emergency Medical Service co-workers and First Responder members are going to run into many personal, work related difficulties and life-changing challenges. I want people to know there is always an option for a better outcome. When you get hurt, broken, depressed and need a friend we are on at your side "no questions asked" for you deserve our love and caring help. When we stand as a team we will show the world we are so worthy of the respect we so deserve. We must also never disrespect our profession as that makes us all just a little less as an entity. Just know and always remember that "**No matter how bad your day is you are never alone.**"

> *At the end of the shift or at the end of your day, I want you to know you matter …*
> *you matter to us all. In the end, I want you to know you all matter…*
> *You matter to me more than I can ever tell you…*
> *You all matter to someone.*
>
> **Dale M Bayliss**

Introduction

There comes a time when we have everything to gain and nothing left to lose in trying to save a life. After all, I would say all life is irreplaceable even if we can't or don't understand why they are present on earth. We often run into people who are not as fortunate as many others, they may live on the streets, many have lost everything but they still value all life. Often, we forget that many people have some very tragic occurrences during their lifetime. Many used to be just like us until something terribly went wrong. Some have even worn a uniform of our very proud military, been police officers, from a fire service, or fellow EMS staff. Tragically somehow, they ended up losing everything. Just know all people have the right to have a terrible time during their lifetime. When we are called to render aid, we need to give them a fighting chance. We need to give them hope. We need to ensure we try our best to turn their life around and head them in the right direction before it is too late.

Somehow, we need to share with all others how important or valuable life should be to everyone. My simple but complex question to you is "Why would my life be any more special than yours?" Maybe ask yourself these questions; Why do people do what they do? or What went so wrong that made their life turn out so depressing or tragic? Then ask yourself simply this final question. "Why did they go from being a normal person to someone living with poor clothing, no real food, no fresh water and no real home?" I would say that everyone has a story to tell if only we could find out the real story just maybe we could help them change their destiny which for many is never good. We can't just pick or choose who we help or why we help them. We need to help anyone in need of our help. Even if it means turning around on a busy day and heading up an unfriendly hill. People are counting on us to do what is right and so is your heart.

I want to show you that by being just the right person in just the right place at just the right time, with the help of the right people, lives can be spared and destiny will be challenged. For many events, I was just the right person or partnered with the right partner to respond to the many unique and challenging lifetime events of people's lives that were in need. When we were called we responded and we worked as a team. We did our best during the call and we helped each other after the call to get our ambulance back in order and then we were ready for the next call, then after our shift we went home as a team. It was a code of honour or a personal code that we needed to master in order to survive. I constantly remind myself that it was never just me that helped people it was the team. Just as I will never forget how much people have helped me get to this part of my career and for that I must never forget it's importance. My destiny was never simply to sit and watch the world go past until my fate was arranged by a higher power.

Many of you will ask the question that is hard to answer to many people in the EMS profession: How do we do it? I'd say it was our destiny just as it was fate that our paths crossed with our patients. I would also say some of us have a greater drive to help others in need than most people. In EMS, many of our members have an inner power that no one can see. Not everyone is cut out to endure our profession for it takes special hard-working people to survive. I would then proudly but quietly say we do it because we can and we do it because people need our help.

Only some of our patients will ever feel or be able to attest to our true powers to save their life. Many may benefit from our actions, for many receive our therapeutic interventions and then receive our ongoing treatments until they arrive at a hospital. Some of our patients were conscious or completely awake and aware of the events around them, possibly aware of their injuries, all while many will not remember us as they were altered in their mental status or fortunate enough to be unconscious in the worst situations. Many won't even know or be able to remember our names. Ironically many will never forget our faces or the sound of our voice after our short but intimate encounter even when they were in shock.

There are also many patients that can't hear us when we are caring for them but will have benefitted from our healing touch in many ways. Even now some can still feel our therapeutic touch on their body. From deep in their heart and even their souls they will have felt us even after they get better for they can still know the love and kindness that came in their time of need and it's the reason they are alive. Life gives life, just as life can take life.

On many occasions, we are the ones that are responsible that gave them more time when time was not an option. Possibly we provided them with just a little extra life when possible and we challenged their destined time or fate when possible. We would not take losing as the only option when we knew they had a reason or a way to live. If it was not their time to leave this planet we kept them alive. We changed destiny when we could, often against the odds that were fighting against us all. When it was meant to be, we made a difference in life and helped the living. When we lost, we still did our best for the patient, their family and their significant others. We treated their lost family members as if they were one of our own.

All our patients had to matter and they would know we didn't choose who we would help. The biggest choice was how hard we worked, how much thought it took to come up with the best strategy to help the sick and the injured and then the amount of effort we made for them to feel they mattered. When we were called, we responded, we assessed and we treated the greatest life threats possible and intervened whenever possible. We came and evaluated our calls, the unique situations, then found the best solution for the current event, overcame the complications and faced the chaos despite the challenges we often faced.

Everyone on our team mattered. The teams were often complex. It started with the first responders, the RCMP or police officers, the firefighters, the BLS crews, the ALS providers, the STARS crews, the critical care transport teams, the receiving hospitals, the physiotherapy and also the pastoral care or grief workers. The list was complex but unique or different in almost every situation. Everyone involved was responsible for the outcomes and for the care of our patients. Many of the same volunteers or our co-workers helped with the survivors, the people affected after the incidents or with the loss of any patient as well.

I was always amazed that one person on our team would often build a personal bond with one patient and make them just a little more special. They would make it their mission to ensure we actually went a little further, worked harder or cared even more than we could or should have. Often for no other reason at all other than they mattered to that one person more than to the rest of the team. That was how emergency medicine often worked in your favour as a patient for you always had one person on your team that cared even more than the others for no real reason other than you mattered. A word of caution to the people who were nasty and hated life it is always best to keep one real friend on your list of people that matter. Being nice has its rewards just as being nasty has its fair rewards as well.

We had our many success stories among them and we had our share of personal tragedies. We often missed the fact that if we counted the ones we lost and compared them to the success stories we still saved thousands and thousands. Somehow that needed to matter to some of us more than others. Very often we relived the bad calls in our mind many times during the day or night when we should have been sleeping. They were truly the unwanted friends that just barged in and wrecked our day. Often smells, sounds, feelings, or similar events triggered them to resurface.

Many people suffering with PTSD would have places they could not go or be present. Often, they would not feel safe in that one specific situation or location for the rest of their career and possibly for life. The best example I can give you all would be "panic attacks" that were common when kids cried or screamed out that would trigger our fight or flight mechanism. Often people with PTSD were triggered by very simple events. I think it's easy to describe, if you think of our body as an egg and the more cracks it gets, the more integrity we lose in our personal structure. Once you have been broken and smashed and your leaking out your precious soul we are never the same again. Many people were affected by the repeated tragedies we were involved in and we often did not realize it until it was too late just how vulnerable people could be as health care workers or EMS providers.

Unfortunately, we never counted the good calls or the ones that really mattered as we were always too critical of our actions on most days. We should have humbly counted when we did save or help the people in need a little more often. Many times, the ones we lost affected us as they were still someone that mattered, but I think they were the ones that proved to us all that we are mortal and that no life is truly immortal. Remember this one line and repeat it often. "Help the ones we can, do your best every day and when we lose we still have done our best." That's what needs to count the most. That's what needs to matter at the end of the day.

The EMS world is not a forgiving world by any means. Sometimes we only get one chance to save a life, so we'd better get it right the first time. Many times, life hangs on a very narrow ledge. One slip or one mistake and they are gone forever. Yet with the right person grabbing hold of their life and making the right interventions, lives are brought back. Suffering is lessened. We were there to help when we could be, and we tried our best. Just know that we responded, we assessed and we identified the threats to life and we intervened as best we could. Every circumstance was unequally different in most presentations. No two calls will ever be the same. No two patients were identically the same, had the same past history or responded the same to our medications. Patients don't always follow the rules of living or how to stay alive. The treatment for one patient may not work for the next. One of the best rules to teach our students or to remind ourselves was to treat your patient and not the monitor on most occasions but not all.

The strange part about emergency medicine was that one intervention for your current patient may not be as effective as it had for the last patient so we needed to be adaptable in our approach to patient care and be able to overcome any complications the best we can in the shortest time we have available. We often measure success by mere seconds or a few valuable minutes. The platinum ten minutes to save a life is so important, whereas the real golden hour from the International Trauma Life Support (ITLS) in trauma care is just a dream for many; it almost never works for the rural EMS care providers. Often, we need different guidelines for urban and rural practitioners to provide holistic care.

When it came to trauma care there were many variable considerations to always consider. If you looked at all the calls we did, often it just came down to fate or possibly bad luck as the deciding factor on saving a life. Sometimes luck is on our side and sometimes it's one hundred and ten percent against us all. For the lucky patients, they got cared for on the receiving side at the local Emergency Rooms (ER) by a trained Advanced Trauma Life Support (ATLS) physician and the injured patients would then have even an increased chance at having a better outcome at the end of what was about to be a terminal end of their day. The further you were away from a trauma surgeon with a stocked blood bank and an available operating room ready to go, increased your chances to do poorly after a major traumatic event. For the fortunate to have a good ground ambulance service, trained rural hospitals with ATLS trained staff and with quick efficient transport protocols in place you too were also blessed.

When we were called we responded often out of nowhere and we would take hold of the many lost or broken soul's. We would grasp onto them as hard as we can and hang on for dear life. Very few people will know our personal strengths and weaknesses except our own EMS team members and the health care workers that we constantly interacted with. Many of the hospital and the support staff we work with twenty-four hours a day will see our personal struggles and also share our success stories. The sickest of the sickest often survived due to the wisdom and the efficiency of the staff in the emergency rooms. They were often the hero's in my EMS world.

Many of the ER staff would gladly receive our patients too, would then help with our failures in trying to help the worst or the sickest patients. Often, we made the patients better before we arrived in the local ER but not always. On some calls nothing went right and we often just could not get everything done before we arrived at the local ER. Hopefully they will not judge us but support us during our bad times. We need to remind each other that no matter how hard we try, we cannot save or help all patients. Sometimes when our patients are suffering or killed it was simply their destiny.

I wonder if they were destined for another stopping point that is just out of our control. All I know is even when we try our best we have bad luck and we are very human. I know that on a bad day I miss my share of intravenous starts, can't seem to intubate easily, or miss the most common signs and symptoms. I just know when we work forty-eight to ninety-six hour shifts, we get tired and are sometimes pushed too far mentally, physically, and emotionally to realize we are in need of being pulled out of service for a needed rest. This would be any and all EMS providers worst kryptonite.

We had a hard time saying no or from being able to just shut off our caring switch.

On the good side, I would have to say we are also special in our ability to save lives. Our unique power is real and the power of our crew is surreal if we add up our feats against so much suffering and personal tragedy. Our personal touch will give life and it will put life into the hearts of others one patient at time. One by one we will make a difference. A few times in my life I've seen and used super feats of strength to save lives. I've also seen miracles. Even if it was just once, it was worth it to the people involved. I was blessed as I was around long enough to see more then one miracle even if I didn't know it right at that exact second of time. But I would still say any patient we helped and made better was a miracle some days, as it was most likely a life saved that should have been lost without our interventions.

We sometimes have to choose who will live and who must die. The art of picking and sorting who we can help the most called *"Triage"* is not as easy as it looks. Some days we would have to trade one life for another, depending on the number of patients we faced and the injuries they had suffered. It was one more reason to not sleep some nights.

We would also need to absorb and treat others' pain and suffering. It's the price of caring for others even if we don't want to and can't easily admit it. The true challenge was to be able to save the ones we can and let the ones we lost go. Simply put, if people didn't matter we could never do this job. There is no amount of money available in the world would help to balance the horrors we see from day to day. I look back and many times I performed the role as the "Triage officer" and it is my cross to bear for I had to choose as required or others would have to unnecessarily suffered or died as well.

After the most tragic calls we too have a grieving period, a time to reflect, but we have to sometimes just sit down and figure out whether we did the right treatment. Every once in awhile, doubt sets in even if we did the right thing. Then we need to move on to the next call and try to always do the right thing again. For most cases, we simply need to let go. Letting go is sometimes the hardest part when we care too much or work so hard trying to save patients. Caring has a high price for many of our EMS workers who develop post-traumatic stress disorder (PTSD), as well as accumulating compassion fatigue, all of which cause early deaths and personal self-destruction.

No one is immune to the pain and no one person in EMS can say that they are okay when they look in the mirror after some of our worst calls. Many times, our local and provincial protocols as well as our limited medications, our limited resources all go against us. The lower we lower the bar the harder our real job comes to the ones that care the most. I just wish we could balance the power bar to make our system better but as with all professions growth is time dependant.

In EMS, we need to be willing to take the chance and make a decision in our patients' care in seconds. More importantly, we need to know in seconds the right pathway to take to achieve the best options for care with the facts we have upon arrival and not simply by following a protocol. We need to know the risk versus the benefit of all interventions and we must be willing to take our best-educated guess. No one can judge us or our actions but a higher power. Many calls don't follow a protocol or any human logic. We simply do our best and see what happens; then we reassess and provide care as required.

Many patients have altered the normal presentations so the standard of care is not appropriate to the point that it's become a big grey area in our emergency medicine world. We have to make a decision and own it despite the outcomes it may create. No one is perfect. No one in EMS has an all-seeing and all-knowing wisdom. When you're dealing with complex medical, surgical and traumatic cases you must deal with the problem even if it's not in your realm of experience.

Life isn't easy for anyone that survives in EMS over the years of service. We work in a complex world. The EMS world attracts the best of the best but also hurts us more than you could imagine. We always want to do the right thing when sometimes the right way doesn't exist. Some days it's a lose-lose situation and it was that way from the start of the call. That's the part that eats away at us in our subconscious. It attacks our sleep and we have bad days even when we have so much to live for that we may not even notice when our world becomes cloudy or dark.

Only a select few will ever know our most sacred secrets but many have felt our healing touch. Sometimes only one person is left at our side when our world crumbles apart and will take our side and back us up when everyone else gives up. Our partners are our real lifesavers – they are our most loyal guardian angels. At the end of the day, all we have is our EMS family to back us up when we are in trouble. A real partner keeps us out of harm's way and from doing harm to others.

No one else will really know our pain but possibly one or two special people. No one else will ever be allowed to enter our hearts and help take away the grief that weakens us from time to time but those select few. No one else will truly be able to understand what roads we've travelled or the difficulty we have faced in order to survive.

Together we the chosen 'lucky' few will change the destiny of others. But as in everything we are only so good for so long and like everything one day we will lose our edge. The hardest part is to know when we are at that point before causing harm. We need to walk away just before that magic day. For many, hopefully your career is just starting and will run as smoothly as possible despite the bumps you will find along the road of life. To you all, I will always consider you my friend. To many, you will forever be my brother and sister in EMS until the end of eternity.

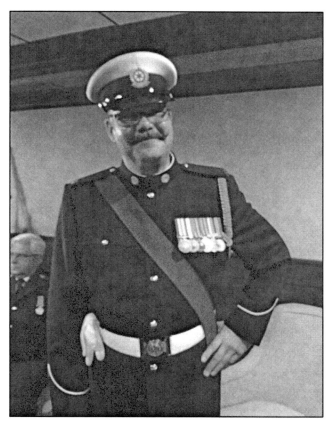

Our Honour Guard

"Anyone that stands for our profession is one of my true heroes."

"The Risk Takers"

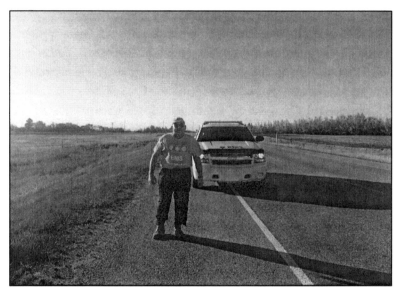

"Challenging Life's Limits"

The "Emergency Medical Services (EMS) world" attracts some very unique and special people. The fact that I made it this long in the EMS field must mean I made the grade, hopefully for all the right reasons. I was attracted to this field of care to help people in need for my personal reasons – that was to just be entitled to help the people in need. Once I found out that there was a need for EMS personnel and they had a vacancy in the profession for some real dedicated good people I dived in head first without even a second thought. Once I got in, I found a huge need for EMS staff members everywhere I travelled, as well as in every community I've lived in. Everywhere I went people were needed in medical care at all levels. Sadly, we will never be unemployed or out of work. Our world sort of keeps creating more and more tragedies despite the technological advances in the world. Somehow society has created a constant increase of drinking and driving, drug abuse and a society that needs to be catered to on multiple levels.

The EMS world has become much more diverse and, as many people forget all too often, we are a new profession. The rest of my career, I would be continually learning and expanding my scope of practice. The personal and systemic challenges of the EMS world would always be very dynamic, physically, mentally and also spiritually challenging. Throughout my story, you will be taken along with us on our emergency calls and, you will see the good side of the profession but you will also see the side that is the most difficult. I will literally take you to hell and then will willingly come to pick you up and bring you back to show you the real reasons why we do what we do for others. In the end, you will realize the world is very connected at all levels. Everyone is connected by some pathway.

You will see pure determination, personal pride and an increasingly complex EMS system that is constantly evolving. I will show you all it is a worthy profession for others to follow if you have just the right stuff. The right stuff is much more than education, much more than endurance and much more than a way of life. You will seem to have the right stuff; you will need to change your way of life and your way of living. You will need to reach deep inside your soul and you will need to give everything you have to change the patient's outcome from something that was bad to something better.

Helping others was one hundred percent my personal choice right from the start of my introduction to the EMS world. Once I got started I simply stood my ground and made my battle against illness, against premature death and fought the human destruction people faced from a bad outcome. I made it my life's mission at all cost. I never realized that there were some parts of our job that were truly the unseen or unknown harmful side effects to us for caring for others. Many don't see the silent but deadly aspects of the job that can also hurt us all even if we don't see it coming until it's too late. They are the effects of Post Traumatic Stress Disorder (PTSD) or maybe more commonly compassion fatigue. This is a mostly misunderstood mental disorder that can occur in certain people after being exposed to traumatic experiences.

Over the years, I would learn many hard lessons – that helping people came with a personal price, despite the rewards. The price was mine to bear and I'd do it again at half the wages, even knowing it would challenge us all to our limits on so many occasions. The tears, the pain and the rewards all made it worthwhile, despite the fact that we are sometimes fighting a losing battle right from the start, which ironically never occurred to me until later in my life.

Looking back at my lifetime experiences I would say that human evolution and changes to such a modern society have not all been for the good. Many changes with new interventions have also brought along more complex issues, and with that additional challenges. The fact that I only know how to help people maybe blinds me to the real world and the negative effect it has on us all. Many issues around us affect us either directly or indirectly. The simple fact we have receptor selective medications now to help people with pain such as fentanyl as an example of the modern advances in medicine and added complex problems to our society.

We started using fentanyl in around 1993 in EMS. But the fact they have now synthesized the medication in home-style laboratories that it's so much more powerful than expected. Sadly, it's now causing a huge strain to all health care systems as well as killing thousands who are not expecting its powerful effects. This makes me wonder if it was a good advancement in such a powerful narcotic to even be worth it at all. This simple one fact or question would cause me many sleepless nights. To know we created a drug that is now a demon, and a huge burden to all levels of EMS, taxing the emergency departments and then also the ICU's, is a real concern many don't see or want to even know about. No amount of naloxone or Narcan® can save a society that will use and abuse any drug they can find to achieve pleasure or a mythical high even if the risk of death is through the next unopened door.

Regardless of the societal demands on us all and my personal struggles with the many people around me, I choose to try and help people in need anyways. When I hurt or I'm having a bad day I still go to work simply knowing I have it much better than many people. My role as a paramedic gives me a specific purpose and not out of necessity in my case. I don't do it just for the money or the gratitude. I do it for the personal satisfaction of being able to help others in need anywhere, anytime and in any crisis 24/7. There is nothing like walking into a disaster, taking charge, finding the problems we can fix, creating a solution to the visible problems and getting the sick or injured to a better place despite the many obstacles. The challenges are unique as well as complex, but the solutions are always in reach if you're able to weigh out your options and create a solution to any event while applying your knowledge. Over time the wisdom from within makes the decisions faster and more accurate then we are given credit for in multiple cases or events.

I have learned by some very influential people to try to always see the good in all people as well as know who was bad and I made sure I stayed away from the bad side of life for a good reason. When I was a kid I made some bad choices but as with everything and everyone, I am human and could learn from my misadventures. In the end, you can appreciate that it's also part of everyone else's life as well. We are all human. Every day at work we all see life has its ups and downs but that's part of living and part of our own evolution as people within mankind.

Many years ago, I decided to give just a little more effort to help others in need and that was just what I did. I would ensure someone was looking out for people in need and we would help them to get to a better place regardless of the obstacles they were facing. I would often push myself to my limits and also enable my friends to do more and more for people that were less fortunate. When working EMS, we would face life's challenges together as a team and help others overcome medical or personal concerns. We would find a solution to all medical or traumatic events when possible for the patient. One at a time we made our patients better off or we helped them to somehow end up in a better place. We would help them when possible to turn around a bad medical situation and come out of a bad place even if it meant it cost us time, our own money or some lost sleep. It as part of what we did best.

We would meet any emergency head-on and find a solution. Even if the solution is not always perfect, it is often better than when we started if at all possible. On most of our calls or cases we performed the right procedure or treatment to make the person better off, but a few times, unfortunately we would make it worse. Very rarely our good intentions would cause more harm than good. That harm we created was many times some of the most monumental teaching or learning points for everyone involved. Nobody in EMS or in health care can claim they always make the right choice for every patient. We all have calls or patients in our past to remind us of our treatment failures. No matter the case or regardless of the outcome we can learn and improve our personal education or learn from our daily adventures.

My personal challenge was to do more than others when it came to alleviating patients' pain, decreasing suffering or smoothing the rocky road they were headed down during a medical emergency.

My dream caught on slowly with others and together we began to have a greater impact on others' lives. Over the years many of my partners and students have carried on my legacy. Often, we take the worst life has to offer in terms of people's health, in life's misfortune, after an accident, and we make life as good as possible for many in the aftermath.

We often risked ourselves physically, mentally, emotionally and spiritually despite the personal challenges we did our absolute best. Along the way, we accumulated some bad emotions or toxic feelings from repeated tragedies that can build and build inside any of us over time. Occasionally, we also got hurt physically, mentally and emotionally despite our personal protective barriers. Sometimes our personal protection equipment (PPE) was completely ineffective. We would get knocked down or taken down with illness or injury just like everyone else. After some very bad outcomes we had nothing left but our desire to carry on and help others, and that was what got us back up.

Sometimes it's the foresight of knowing the outcome if we could not carry on that picked us up when we got knocked down so hard. A very good saying is if we fall seven times we must get up eight times. Sometimes knowing the outcomes for our patients without interventions pushes us even harder to defeat the fate or destiny they might have had in the end. We sometimes got back up and fought even harder because knowing the outcomes would be devastating if we looked the other way or ignored people's difficulties. Many of us assumed our patients' battle to live and we fought destiny and fate all at the same time. Once you've started to fight for a patient we assumed the role to keep fighting the battles for life until it was over for better or worse. Regardless of the type of problems, we fought and challenged every chance complications imaginable.

If someone was in big trouble or in hell and needed a rescue we simply went and got them. Then we literally pulled them back out without ever needing to know the how or the why they got there in the first place. We would simply try to fix any medical complication despite the reasons, no matter how it occurred. Matt Anderson's song "Bold and Beaten" says it better than I could ever do. It simply says, *"Little girl. I'll follow you down, I don't know how far we go, I need to see you get your feet on the ground, you don't need to tell me. I don't need to know."* That song is so truthful in my opinion. It makes my heart warm up knowing we can actually stop and help others in need, regardless of the reasons it's simply a start.

Most times when people get knocked down in life it's just part of the day. But some days you get hit so hard it makes the getting up that much harder. I can honestly say I have seen a side of hell that many of our patients end up being knocked down too. More than once we tried to save many patients from a very bad outcome and it was worthy of the cost in every separate occurrence. If you think of the hundreds we have brought back from being in a very unstable medical situation or traumatic event, it is truly amazing. Even if we just saved one or two out of the hundreds, it would be worth it to me for all our attempts were never in vain. Only a few times did I actually get hurt or cut up by some crazy person or work-related injury. Thankfully, after a bad day, my golden retrievers, my close friends, my fellow co-workers and my physician friends have always been my backup. With no regrets, they often fixed me or sutured me up after every time when I was hurt in the line of duty. They were more than happy to make my day better and I can't think of one episode where they didn't go out of their way to treat me just a little more special for just doing my job. They are the best of the best. They will be my personal friends for life.

On shift or our workdays, we always become a team. No matter what our similarities or differences are, we make it work. Every shift we simply work as a team to provide the best possible care to our patients. Only rarely did I need to step in to rescue my partner from harm but it did happen. A few times my partners also stepped in and saved me from harm as well. We had the rule that if a patient was pushing the wrong buttons and making us angry, we would do our best to switch out if possible. Sometimes we could avert a conflict but sometimes our clientele were just bad and nothing could ease the discomfort of trying to deal with them on good terms.

Thinking back, every once in awhile, I had no choice but to step in and take someone else's pain or injury if a bad person was going to harm one of my co-workers. We sometimes went to many extremes to help people from time to time even when it was not our fight or our battle. If you saw a fellow EMS member in trouble, you made their problem your problem. If one of us needed help, they were our first and only priority. Looking back, some of the times were just a little bit crazy but regardless of the call or the situation, we went and performed our best just the same despite the consequences. In the end, we always made it back despite the rather complex situations we faced. Being a team member had its privileges I would honestly need to say. If you were on my team you stayed on the team. If you disrespected us or disgraced us, you were taken off the team. I always gave people a chance but after they had one chance and they blew it, I was done with helping them.

It was always rewarding when you looked back at how hard staff would work to save the life of a complete stranger. Many times, we would try harder than humanly possible. This was us simply knowing that a worse outcome for others exist for all of our patients without divine intervention. If we knew our patients or they were one of us, we worked even harder. With experience, we would attempt to abort some bad outcomes as soon as we realized that we could intervene in a quicker fashion to abort or prevent a bad or worse outcome in many cases when possible. It was alike to a guard dog watching over a flock of innocent helpless creatures.

The pending threat to our patient's lives can push us to work harder and harder to make sure that their lives were spared. From time to time we will even be required to assume more potential risk, for we know sometimes people don't get a second chance in life in certain life-threatening circumstances. If we could identify a life threat we neutralized it when possible. We simply headed it off and changed our patient's destiny without a single second of hesitation.

Despite seeing the worst of the worst, we got up the next day and faced life's challenges with vigour like it was a new day, for that is exactly what it was to me. We went to work and faced the challenges we could see and attempted to steer our patients in the right direction when possible to ensure the best outcomes are achieved. We can't always change destiny but we can always challenge it and we don't quit until we've run out of all known options. Many of us take losing personally and we learn from life's lessons to ensure we do better next time. After all, saving lives and helping people is an art and the skills required are mastered only with time and wisdom. Nobody gets it right every time. Nobody is perfect. No one on earth is perfect as far as I can see or from what my limited view on the millions of people from around the world has demonstrated. I truly only can say that I have more faults then many others so I have no right to judge others at any time.

My life of helping people has left me with nothing to complain about other than a few small but meaningful regrets. The biggest regrets are simply that we missed helping some of our own people along their troubled roads. We lost them to missing facts or the subtle clues that they were in hell and we never got the message until it was too damn late to rescue them. Losing a partner or a friend in EMS hurts more than most to many of us. When you have put your life on the line with your partner and you have worked with someone so hard to save a life and then one day they take their own life it is a indescribable pain. It is breath stopping or heart breaking to suddenly realize we missed the signs of the life threatening trouble that would haunt us for the rest of our life. In the end, after it is all said and done, you realize they have prematurely taken their own life; it hurts.

We were put in this world to help people but the question we forgot to think about was simply: "Who helps us when we get broken?" Sometimes there is no right answer. If we asked for help we would most likely get it now, but not in the past. Mostly we were just too proud or possibly too scared to ask. We just ignored the pain and over time we lost the battle with pain and internal suffering and we will come face to face with PTSD. I was one of these people and it is only recently I could admit it. Regardless of the sanctions against me I stand and fight for the right cause. I'm not embarrassed to say it hurts to lose from time to time, even if many times we win.

The losses build up and go against us for we are perfectionists at heart and losing is not in in our list of acceptable options. I think we will find out our situation of always being around the hurt and injured actually puts us in a more complex form of PTSD that is not understood at all by our present mental health staff, our current family physicians, our EMS managers and by anyone else involved in health care.

Please don't get me wrong because we have many rewards for helping people. The bad calls are not very often but when they come they affect us all. The personal satisfaction we receive is the biggest reward for anything we do for others. The best thing is to look for the good things and that keeps me from seeing the negative world around us most days. The news always seems to cover the bad things; there is not much of a reward for providing the world with good news. My personal choice is not to watch TV or read the highlights as the bad stuff is repeated 24/7. The negative events on TV are not a fair picture of the real-world local, regional or national events. We need to see the good in our lives, and we need to look for the good in others as well.

The good things should count the most for all of us. I know everything I need that is good in life and anything I need is in my grasp if I want to receive it. If I can see it and it's good for me, it's mine for the right price and adequate effort. Nothing I need is unreachable.

Our goals and personal ambitions are normally attainable. Sadly, we will never run out of patients, so we will never be unemployed. This world has ensured we will always have endless work; even if we could prevent certain accidents or specific diseases we just can't seem to change our course in life. So, in the end it's always a good and bad day for many people regardless of our effort.

My past education and my experience has helped me to face the challenges we see from day to day. I'm actually more than ready and willing, at least in my mind, to go on the calls with my partner. The times I'm not working are the harder times. I repeatedly would think back to calls and many times I debate the choices we made; and it always brings up some form of doubt. Just imagine if you were working with us and we had three separate serious calls and for each call you went out of your comfort zone. This is easy when you're treating someone and you have no clear idea of the internal problems.

We are sometimes guessing, only to find out we were wrong after arrival at the local ER. Among all the bad calls we had one cardiac arrest that was an unsuccessful resuscitation, all while you're still trying to figure out the first call of the day. Then we also had three separate, horrible motor vehicle collisions (MVC)s over the last week with one-person dead and then three more patients in critical condition. Your week went from bad to much worse. When you can imagine that, then you're walking in our shoes even if it's just as an observer. It still counts.

That alone shows our life isn't always easy. We simply finished one call and went to the next one without debate or question. Only my partner really noticed my tears and she told no one, as she was crying too but that was our little secret. We both never had enough time to grieve or to stop long enough to gather our thoughts to a better place. There were days the calls kept coming and we kept responding. Even when we thought we had nothing left, my partner smiled at me and together we acknowledged the next call, as we were always a team. It was the team spirit that kept us going. Nothing else mattered.

Every one of those calls affected multiple people: the families, the friends, the EMS involved, the police, the victim services all the way to the STARS staff and don't forget the pilots. The staff at the local funeral homes, the chaplains and pastors must have cried themselves to sleep that week. The guardian angels could not keep up with us despite using wings and working in teams twenty-four hours a day and seven days a week. It was a battle no one could have won on their own. Our actions or lack of actions affect everything we do on a call or with our patient care. Even if we had no hope of saving the lost, we still tried our best and prayed we could have made a bad outcome a little better when possible. It was sometimes not to be and heaven or another world needs people too, so we had to let some go, despite not being willing to say goodbye.

I have over thirty-five years working the streets saving lives, helping others and trying to make the world a better place. I have my overall health, but the aches along with the heartbreaks are always there and they are very real. I still can move and function well and when needed I can move very fast but sometimes I'd rather not be wearing a lifesaver's cape and simply not be needed so much. After years of seeing sick and dying people, you accumulate more than you need and you simply want to walk away from the EMS life. I will never be rich but I have money in the bank when it's needed. I have food in the fridge and a place to call home. The song lyrics "Bold and Beaten" come to mind right now. The four lines from Matt Anderson's song says it so well in my case:

> *"I'm alone, but I'm not lonely*
> *I've got friends everywhere I go*
> *I've got a house, but still no home*
> *I take shelter in my songs."*

My current home is more of a stopping place in my life to enable me to sleep and hangout with my precious golden retrievers Pebbles and Tinsel until I can move on and get to where I want to end up in life. It is safe and meets my needs so it serves its purpose well. I have a place to rest and a place that's safe for my animal family members. They actually like it more than I do. I'm sure it's set up for them to have extra luxury, not for me. Someday I will have my dream house facing the ocean and be able to appreciate the sound of true silence. Then I will have inner peace and my life will be complete.

My retirement home will enable me to wander along in life and have no schedule other than walking along the ocean and watching the tide cycle around the moon's schedule is fine with me. I know that my golden retrievers will love the open water as they love to swim and play outside. They can swim every day so long as they don't mind the cold water in the winter and yes, I will be at their side just to keep them safe. Tinsel was always a water dog and thankfully she taught Pebbles how to swim. Teamwork in all lives is very important. My goldens took the word team to an all time better description.

My home is very basic and relatively quiet. The kids have all moved out and they are on their own, working to make their own identities unique, so that is a good thing. I have my two golden retrievers Pebbles, Tinsel and two undercover cats that kill little four-legged rodents that I hate in or around my house. Someday I might just find the right person who can put up with my work ethics and my crazy life but if not, I keep walking ahead in life. I will work as hard and as long as possible, ignoring my pain and continue to fulfill my need to help others more than myself. This will go on until I can't give my one hundred and ten percent anymore. Then I will walk away from it all, on my own terms.

My whole life has been on my terms and that is the way it must be but just as the little guy in the movie "Angels in The Outfield" would most often say, "It could happen." In the end, I will look after what happens in my life as and I will live with my EMS and hospital family members as my real family. They are the ones that matter so much to me. We will somehow face the daily challenges, accept the personal and work related events after what ever happens just "happens" as our lives unfold.

Looking back and knowing what I know now I would have to say that I'm not surprised when our Guardian Angels suffer from a broken wing, or suffer from a broken spirit from seeing what we see . When you work so close to real danger you're bound to get hurt from time to time.

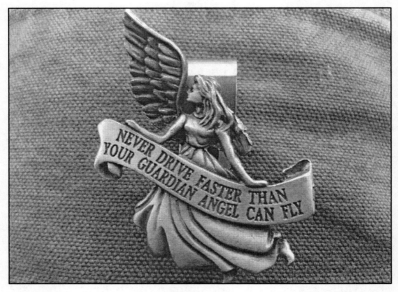

Guardian Angels

"In EMS, Health Care, or as First Responders, even when we are broken or injured we will always try to do our best."

Chapter 2: Setting the Stage for Success
"My EMS Family and More"

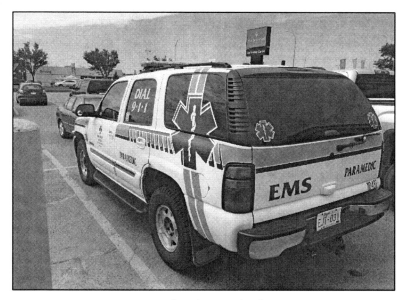

AHS "Modern Backup"

Lisa was my full-time EMS partner and had been my best partner for my whole career in the EMS industry. I could not find a better emergency medical technician (EMT-A) or a better working partner in this whole big round world. She was only registered as an EMT-A but was as wise as most paramedics I've worked with in the past. We were working our first day shift and it was not my favourite shift, as we both enjoyed night shifts much more. Night shift just had far less politics than most of the day shifts. Nights have always been my personal favourite, as they tend to be the most challenging, with some of the strangest and/or hardest calls. Some night shifts turn into very long days. With the right partner, the shift was tolerable no matter the dangers, no matter the hardships we would have prevailed them all as a team.

Sadly, the night shift will also bring out the worst evil that hides in the true darkness of the night. We all know and have learned the hard way that the worst evil hides in the people of the night. The majority of our most violent crimes tend to occur in the middle of the night or in the early hours of the morning. The days are most likely when the bad people are sleeping and dreaming up ways to cause more harm and grief to the unfortunate or unlucky. Most nights, the good people are sleeping in the safety of their home, and most have no idea of the shady nightlife around us all. The sleeping population has no idea of the number, and extent of the atrocities or the badness that occur sometimes just a few doors away from them while they are sleeping. Most good people are trying to recharge for another honest day of work to come. Only a select few will be awakened by the badness hiding in the darkness. This is when our friends the RCMP or police forces earn every cent that they make defending our lives sometimes at the cost of their own lives.

The unlucky EMS staff, the health care staff, the firefighters and the many police working shift work get to see the consequences of the evil people that affect others in negative ways. When we all work together we greet the challenges from every call and handle it the best we can as a team. Somehow, we find a way to make the broken systems function better and we conquer every situation despite the often-limited resources.

The real team is the EMS, police, fire, and hospital staff that are always involved in helping the sick, the injured and the broken. We as a team perform miracles whenever possible and when it's not, we do our best and let destiny decide the fate of our patients. After all, we can't change destiny but we can avert many disasters with our wisdom, our team approach and sometimes we had even a little luck on our side.

Regardless of the time of day, when the call comes in, we get to respond. We are thrilled to go out on calls. Not all our staff is as anxious to be paged to go to work, as we are most days. Thankfully I'm a paramedic with a huge knowledge base and have kept up with the educational changes in our industry over time. I have been fortunate to help save thousands of people over the years. I really don't know what it's like *not* to help others. Basically, I've never known anything except pagers or radios, making our days exciting and challenging as well as rewarding. Our extra adrenalin rushes or the excitement does not always help us to sleep after a shift but it is a big part of the job.

No matter how bad the shift was, as soon as I got home my golden retrievers are always waiting at the door. I have had two spoiled dogs that make the worst shift memories go away within seconds of coming in the front door. Pebbles (The Wolf) is eleven years old and her smaller sidekick is Tinsel (The Terminator), is just seven years old. They somehow take away the crap and remove the evil that we see and accumulate internally while at work. They give out so much love they nullify most of the evil from me within mere seconds when they get a chance. Once I get into the safety of my home I'm their responsibility to keep safe. They would take their job very seriously.

One strange fact is that my animals don't know the meaning of a "bad day." As soon as they see or hear my truck in the driveway they are at the window or the door, making the evil run like hell from the inside of me. No one gets past them without permission, or teeth will be displayed. Pebbles, the oldest and toughest, is also the biggest, the real guardian of my home. She has a growl that would scare the already dead. I'm sure she has even scared my kids a few times when they showed up after midnight. That was the latest the puppies would receive visitors. They are the gatekeepers of my home 24/7.

They also give out a special healing light and helped to remove the darkness we are forced to see over and over at work. I eventually learned that no matter how often we see the bad things at work, it always affects us even when we don't think it does. Even if we don't realize it, our work becomes part of us and can corrupt our inner soul over time after many or just one tragic events. We often miss the fact that it truly was a terrible situation as we are too close to the situation to see the bigger picture.

When we are called out we will do our best and try as hard as possible to help people but sometimes we were destined to lose the battle and must let nature and/or destiny do the rest. That is the part we have the most trouble accepting and it's a universal problem in all health fields, police forces, military and firefighters worldwide. We need more Pebbles and Tinsel teams worldwide to reduce the effects of tragedies to our inner self. They might just be one of the best therapies to defeat PTSD or compassion fatigue head on if you consider the options. Unconditional love sometimes has a way to overcome most forms of pain or evil.

Looking back for many years, when I got home, the golden retrievers would suck out the worst memories and throw them out with the trash. It was never recycled. Just by giving unconditional love the bad slowly disappears over the minutes sharing their special hearts with mine. But then suddenly the nightmares and sleepless nights came back. They slowly started coming back bit-by-bit and I just tried to ignore it. But over time I knew it would not go away and slowly I got scared of my past calls. I saw it affected me in ways I never thought possible but thankfully, I had some people in my corner that would fight for my right to live. If it weren't for the right people, in the right place of time and place, I too would have had a bad outcome. I learnt partners were everything to me and when we had each other at our side, we were invincible. We became one and we never left each other's side other than for bathroom breaks during the tour of duty. It is the unique world of having a working partner in life.

Our partners got to know our personal favourites better than anyone. Lisa had just grabbed us a quick coffee from the Timmy's drive-through, which was my personal favourite and my day was somehow complete now. No matter what happened the rest of the shift I had some coffee in me so I could now face the world. We went to Timmy's so often that the staff knew our birthdays and our drink orders as soon as we walked through the door or entered the drive through. They also knew me so well they knew my puppies by name.

Nothing else can make the day start off better than a real coffee with one honey (to fight viruses) and one sugar (for added energy). Some days that initial coffee was lifesaving for it woke me up and it was that first cup that had saved my life daily. It was also lifesaving by giving me a quick drink of a little liquid courage. Then Lisa added more sunshine – even if it was only temporary, it helped. I never had a better partner than Lisa in my whole career. Without her my life would have been terrible on some of my worst shifts.

Lisa has been an EMT for over fifteen years and we have been partners for as long as we both could remember. Lisa is the gentlest lady in the world and has the gift of bringing joy to our day. Over the years, we only find a few gifted people out in the EMS world that do this job for fun, not for the money, and she is one of them. Lisa is the right person for this job. She is the perfect partner for me for as long as my career takes me. Lisa covers for me when I can't give 110% for I have nothing left. She takes over for me on my bad days, especially on the days when I'm so tired I have nothing left to give.

She always has my back and I always have hers. No matter what happened, it was a team effort on or after the end of our shift ended.

We would never ever throw each other under the bus. We always paid special attention to each other and ensured no one else was trying to hurt either one of us. We would always watch each other's back on every call. We also ensured we never missed anything from the dispatch history, to the scene assessment onto the patient assessment. Then while providing care or during our interventions it was always a team effort. It was never wrong to speak your mind or to simply state what you could see or what we were thinking. That's what made our team even better at providing patient care. We each could see a call from a different perspective.

I love my EMS job and I don't often have bad days but once in awhile they creep up and get me when others aren't looking. I remember many of the dead children, the teenagers, the hangings, the abused patients, and the terrible overdoses, and then the people shot or stabbed for some stupid reason. They are all part of the pain and seeing them lying dead in the ER after a code was called often comes back to haunt everyone involved. They are never just forgotten. At one time, they were someone's loved ones. They too mattered.

Every one of them mattered to one of us for some reason and we tried our best to make a difference. Even when we lost the battle to save them we still tried, despite the mortal injuries, we still tried, we still cared. They bring us to tears from time to time and cause an aching pain that won't stop. Sometimes they take away our peaceful dreams on more nights than we want to admit. Our sleep is never really ours when we are on shift or on call but it's the price we gladly pay in exchange to being able to help others in need.

We have the perfect dream job with rarely a dull minute; even on a quiet shift something always happens. Our schedule is somewhat demanding but very rewarding on a ninety-six hour stretch. We work two ten-hour day shifts and then two fourteen-hour night shifts. We often alternate between attending the calls or driving, often depending on whether it's an Advanced Life Support (ALS) call or a Basic Life Support (BLS) call. If it's an ALS call, I often get very busy giving multiple medications or performing advanced treatments. Often, time goes quickly for both of us during a normal shift. Thankfully we never argue about who drives or who attends, as it just happens. If Lisa wants me to attend, I attend. If I need help, Lisa pulls over and we do what we need to. No matter what the problem was, we faced it together.

Everyone loves the real ALS calls as they keep our senses sharp and our minds alert, always expecting a patient's status to change or create a challenge. We expect the ups and downs of our patient's condition so that we can intervene even before the crisis presents itself. We have the ability to know when trouble is just around the corner and we have the knowledge and training to manage that trouble head on. Despite the challenges, I have never regretted the pain and suffering it might have cost me. For most calls, we don't have regrets but we sometimes have trouble forgetting or have the odd nightmare that will never go away for a select few calls. Many nights I wake up thinking about a call and wonder if we could have done better than we did. Many other nights I cannot sleep due to other bad calls. ALS has its benefits but also takes its toll on many people. If we care, it will eventually catch up with us and that is okay as long as we learn to handle the consequences before they cause permanent damage.

Our unit was equipped with the best of the most modern equipment available. We were working in Medic-One and it was a tank on wheels. We had the ability to fly through the night and, so far, Lisa and I had avoided every close call that could have wrecked our day and made our unit history. We take extra pride in keeping our unit cleaned and stocked, and there was always over half a tank of fuel in our ambulance while we were on our shift and it was always full at the end of our shift.

We made sure that the crew that took over our unit was ready to respond to any event. After a call, it was hard to get everything cleaned and the restocking done but it was a very important aspect people never took for granted. Thankfully after a bad call the other crews as well as management staff almost always took time out of a busy day to help us. It showed me they cared and it was also a form of debriefing that made sure we were in the right mindset to carry on with our shift. We had our share of bad supervisors that hid when it was time to work and thankfully they found employment someplace else. After the bad calls, we simply needed each other more than words could ever express.

We worked for one of the busiest services in the province. On average, we did twelve to twenty-four calls per tour, which was enough to keep our skills sharp. I had never had it better in my EMS life, yet I felt something was missing. I knew that whatever it was, it was important but couldn't see what it was nor could I touch it. I didn't know if it was real and I couldn't describe it to anyone else. All in all, my life was never going to get much better so I smiled and kept my head held up high. I was content to do my best; the calls just kept coming and we handled them as we always did. No one could complain about our patient care. We did our best and that was that. Giving less than one hundred percent was not an option. But still something was missing from me even if I could not know what it ever was.

Our daily unit, Medic-One, was a reliable Demeres Ambulance Model 170, one of the toughest units on the road. With a neat interior design and details that contribute to it being a safe, smart workplace to save lives in, we were happy. They have come so far in making ambulances over the last thirty years – from a van, to a truck chassis, to a real complete unit. Our Medic-One was the best in our EMS world. It was the state of the art portable patient care office. When all hell was breaking apart it was always best to get our patient in the unit, initiate care and also to initiate transport to the most appropriate hospital.

We have Medic-Three as backup on our day shifts and Medic-Five as our night shift backup. During normal shifts, our service uses ALS units as backup but when staffing is bad, a basic life support (BLS) unit is our backup. Most days our backup crew is heading towards our location long before being dispatched officially. We have each other's back and that is essential to survival in the EMS world. Without the teamwork and protection of our partners we would not last long in the industry.

We were fortunate in some ways, as we seldom did every inter-facility transfers unless ALS was really needed. Basically, we just responded to emergency calls, fire standbys, accidents, or other trauma injuries, and yes, we did the common medical calls. We do many BLS or basic trivial medical calls, but all-in-all if we are called, we are going to be transporting a patient unless it is decided that transport is not needed. Our life is never dull doing the emergency calls but, unknown to me, my days ahead were going to crumble before my very own eyes. My life and my partner's destiny were not as planned out as we hoped it would have been in the near future. Destiny or fate was in charge of our lives even if we ignored the suggestion that our EMS world would alter, for it was part of the big picture. We just could not see it coming, which all in all was for the best.

If you had asked me I would have said I had about eight years until retirement and would not have even given it a second thought. But unknown to me, my life was going to change. Nothing can and nothing could stop the inevitable. Destiny has plans and forgot to inform me of the pending changes. I just kept heading forward, unaware that trouble was coming right for me and that my life would be changed forever change for good. So often we will do not know until it's too late the extent that just how much destiny or fate will directly and indirectly affect our lives. The people around us should never be taken for granted. We don't know if they will get to see a tomorrow just as we may not make the night.

Our destiny was meant to take us down a certain road. Even though we had no idea of our final destination, we just kept going. I wonder if our pathways are meant to be altered by our past interactions with others. Just as Papa Joe said in the movie "Unconditional," "It ain't a dead end if it takes you somewhere you needed to go." Life knows the road much better than we can ever comprehend. So just remember to always admire the scenery on the roads we travel, as we may never pass this way again. The challenges and the risks we take alter our pathways and inevitably change our direction down life's many pathways. We need to build our character and then stand and defend it as life throws us personal challenges. It's the outcome of the challenges that defines our true character.

My Golden Rule – For Me and My Patients

"Sometimes we will need to bend the rules to save a life, but we should not break our moral code, destroy our ethics, or lose our soul along the way."

Dale M. Bayliss

Dale and Robyn

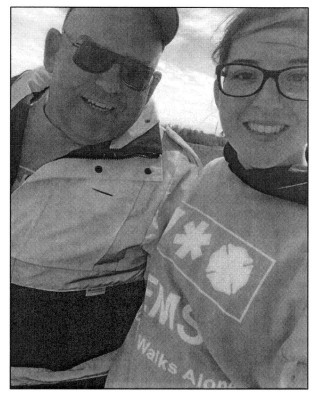

"Making Everyone Count"

Chapter 3: My Baby Is Dying

"Please Help My Baby"

Love knows no real limits

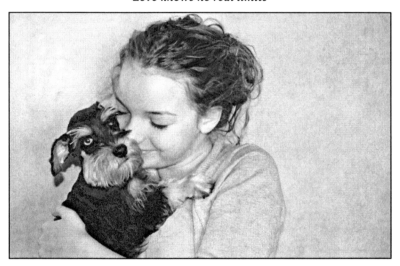

"Little Ones Count More"

The first day shift has been busy but manageable. We have already been to three medical calls this morning. Lunch is not looking like it will happen despite the fact we were both starving for some real food. Today even junk food or fast food is looking better by the hour. Thank God, we both had our morning coffee and it is lasting for a bit longer than it normally would. Our tour has been fun even if the calls have not been too stressful or challenging, not that I always want exciting challenging calls but it makes our day a real challenge.

Regardless, every call was still a good one so we were never bored. Today we have "Ken" as a ride-along and we've been showing him the ropes on how we do real emergency calls. This was while we were trying to talk him into taking the next emergency medical responder (EMR) course ASAP. Then he could register at Keyano College and take the next emergency medical technician – ambulance (EMT-A) course. There are other good schools in the province but this was one of the better ones and if it was good enough for my daughter, it was good enough for Ken.

I'm really old school when it comes to names and definitions so the recent professional title changes from EMT-A to primary care paramedic (PCP) are still a challenge. I still prefer to call them simply "EMTs" with no disrespect intended. I guess I'm so old I won't likely change my terms until the day after I retire. I'm thankful most people now know today we aren't just "ambulance drivers" anymore. More and more of our members are getting degrees, master's and a select few have a PhD in education but sadly not in critical care or in EMS. Our profession is slowly evolving towards self-autonomy but it's taken almost fifteen years. The new graduates are slowly realizing they are the future leaders. They are the ones who will need to push our profession, as I'm out of energy to make our world evolve much more.

The good thing about our job in EMS is we get to help mostly good people. We deal with the bad people too, but only for a short time. By allowing a ride-along we get to see the good people who are trying to get into the EMS industry and we can help them with the application process. In a heartbeat, I can see Ken is one hundred and ten percent good stuff although he's only eighteen years old. He has the right stuff, very polite and caring. A good example of his character was seen on the last call when I saw him smiling and comforting a grandma who had just lost her husband of fifty-seven years. It almost made me cry but I was smiling at the same time. So far, Ken has his First-Aid and American Heart and Stroke "BLS" which is equivalent to the Health Care Provider CPR training. All he needs now is his Class 4 driver's license to be ready for the EMT class as soon as he gets the EMR course completed. With a quick criminal record check at the local police department, he should be ready for any EMS class.

We were dispatched "Code 3" for an eight-month-old infant in distress. All the dispatcher could make out was crying in the background and a frantic "my baby is dying." The sound picked up by the experienced dispatcher thinks the call sounded more like an acute breathing problem, but it's unclear and it was a poor connection. The backup unit and the police are also dispatched as precaution. The caller's phone quit after the call was initiated and the dispatcher got no answer when he called back. The dispatch information is vague and it could be almost anything.

En route, we were both mentally preparing to deal with whatever presented itself. I give Ken some pointers and Lisa looks over and smiles back at me as she's driving high speed with the emergency lights and sirens activated. She's always looked after my back and I have hers. We will both have Ken's back today and ensure he is looked after on all levels. Ken would be kept safe between us no matter what happened. We are advised to use extreme caution by the dispatcher. Our personal and protective shields are up and we ensure our staff is always safe prior to any patient care needs.

We went over the arrival plans, as we got closer to the scene. Lisa was to grab the airway kit, which has the oxygen administration equipment as well as a D-Tank of oxygen and anything needed for immediate airway control. Ken will grab the LifePak-15 (LP-15) cardiac monitor, which has everything, needed to prove signs of life. I will grab the paediatric ALS bag and the ALS drug kit. We are ready for a battle, but until we arrive on the scene we don't know what we will face.

The battles we faced were almost completely unknown on this call. It will be assessing a patient as a team, then attacking the body system in trouble and challenging that system to get with the program and become normal again. Then it will ultimately be to save a life either on scene, in the back of the unit or on the way to the local ER, all in a timely fashion. Losing a kid is not an option, so it was not even a thought that crossed my mind. I was happy we had an extra pair of hands and this will show Ken what BLS and ALS care is in real time.

In the past, we have been to this row of low-income housing many times. We have seen anything from child-abuse cases, to multiple stabbings, to beatings as well as the death of a child with multiple homicides in the same area. We are trying to be mentally prepared and ready for anything, which is not easy. I'm getting very nervous even though I don't say a thing. The backup unit is about a minute behind our arrival on scene, which is very reassuring on unknown calls. Backup on serious pediatric calls is always essential and the extra help is never turned away when it's available. Our standing rule is if it's something that can be done in the house, then it will be done but if the scene is questionable, the little one will be moved to the unit and the resuscitation or the code can be run there, which is often much safer for everyone. I was trying to picture in my mind the most likely complications in today's call but there were too many differential diagnoses to narrow it down without more information. We just need to wait and pray we can handle it on arrival.

As we pull up in our unit, the first RCMP member crew is already on scene. We parked so we could leave immediately if necessary and grabbed our equipment before running into the house, still unsure of what emergency was awaiting our arrival. As we entered the apartment an RCMP officer doing CPR while walking towards us cradling the young child met us at the entrance of the bedrooms. "Shit," I caught myself saying aloud and yelled at my other partners, "Let's just go to the unit!" I helped the RCMP member out of the apartment and down the stairs so he didn't fall and cleared his pathway directly to the unit. As the little one is laid down on the centre of the stretcher it is now our responsibility.

The RCMP member is dripping with sweat as he has worked very hard and efficiently to save a life. I immediately took over the airway care with a quick insertion of the right sized oropharyngeal airway (OPA) to open the little airway past the tongue, then grabbed a small bag valve mask (BVM) with an oxygen reservoir to ventilate the little lungs until the chest started to rise, then I stopped squeezing the little BVM. Ken was ready to take over from the RCMP member on chest compressions. Ken had taken CPR a few times but had never seen it done. He got right in as he was not going to just sit and watch this one play out, for he was now part of the team. Ken had never done CPR for real on anyone so we both coached him along and he was doing his job perfectly. Lisa immediately applied the cardiac monitor, along with the Sp02 and the pediatric end tidal C02 nasal prongs. Lisa then took over, making sure Ken was also okay.

Ken was doing very good chest compressions so we let him continue. The end-tidal carbon dioxide, also known as the ETC02, was rising which told us the CPR was effective. The Sp02 was slowly coming up which is also a great sign of good respiratory and cardiovascular response. The officer quietly stated, "It sure looks like a child-abuse case," speaking to no none in particular. That is when I noticed new and old bruising and swelling on the left side of the child's face and to the chest region. This call just got much harder emotionally for everyone.

On his arrival, the RCMP officer said he found the house a complete mess and had found the child on the floor in a bedroom. There was some blood on the floor and the child was poorly clothed. The parent or caregiver was frantic but also acting completely strange, so they have her in custody. They suspected drug abuse at this time. He said the child was still "gasping" and had ineffective breathing, so he started CPR and that's when we met him while walking towards us. It may sound easy but it's a skill and it was obvious that this member had seen his share of pediatric emergencies. I thought by the way he was looking after the infant he was most likely in EMS but I didn't get the time to ask that simple question. As soon as he was free to use his radio he was calling his dispatch centre asking for more backup. In seconds, his partners will arrive and assist us all in the investigation and protection of this little one in the days to come. The teamwork displayed today was better than just good.

In no time, I was bagging very small amounts of oxygen-rich room air at a slow precise rate and we were artificially breathing for the infant through a very small bag valve mask (BVM). Thankfully I saw the chest rising equally, but I swore again as I found some signs of old and new bruising to the anterior chest and then I could see that one arm is deformed and swollen. I swear to myself and start to shake my head in disgust. Lisa just touched my arm and said nothing. That touch told me I was not alone in my thoughts. Child-abuse cases are hard for everyone to deal with and it gives us all bad feelings for days to come.

Unexpectedly, in a few minutes of CPR we now have a slow weak pulse present, but the chest compressions are still needed because the pulse is too slow to perfuse the infant's body and brain adequately. This little one is essentially in cardiac arrest. The most likely cause is from an airway or breathing complication but an acute head injury could also be the origin of the complication. We will assess the temperature and blood sugar and evaluate the rest of the infant as quickly as we can after we ensure the airway; breathing and circulation "ABCs" are stable and adequate.

I looked up and I could tell the RCMP member was super pissed off. I'm sure his blood pressure (BP) was too high and was rising due to anger but he kept his control almost too well. I know he has young kids at home and that always makes this type of call hurt even more. I know that these calls push us all to our limits mentally, physically and emotionally. Even when we try to control it, it's still not easy. I slapped him on the back and said; "Good job" and I meant it. I could see him acknowledge my appreciation and I knew he was okay despite being so angry with the current situation. This officer had just saved a child and we were his backup. Today the EMS and police services worked as one and a life was pulled from the angel of death. We knew the real outcome was days away but at least now we had something to work with, so that is the blessing of the day so far.

In no time, more police and the backup unit arrived on the emergency scene. We made a game plan and got the second crew to call the dispatch centre and link in the critical care staff to see if they can arrange a pediatric intensive care unit (PICU) transport team to come to our local hospital right away or ASAP. Most likely STARS rotary air ambulance will bring the PICU team right away, as this is the fastest means of obtaining more specialized medical care for the infant. They will most likely bring a pediatrician or STARS doctor who is trained in all types of emergency care, not just what's written in a medical textbook. However, we could still be looking at an hour before the team arrived so we decided it's best to transport to the local ER. They are the best bet for our backup as it's a short transport time and they have the doctors that will help stabilize the infant until the PICU team arrives. Anything that can be done is best done for this little one in the local emergency room (ER) with the efficient and dedicated emergency doctors and nurses. Most of the staff in the ER are trained in PALS and have many years of experience to help make this outcome the best it can be despite the initial presentation.

The LP-15 is on and the heart rate is only about 40 beats per minute (bpm) when chest compressions are paused, which is not fast enough in my mind or by any standards. Most kids if it's less than 60 bpm we simply augment our care along with proper chest compressions along with meticulous airway management. Thankfully it's a sinus bradycardia instead of an idioventricular or asystole rhythm which would have a much worse outcome in the end. Bradycardia in kids is almost always related to hypoxia or hypovolemia and we fix them as quickly as possible with good Basic Life Support (BLS) skills. The oxygen saturation is saying that the Sp02 is now 100% with the positive pressure ventilations (PPV) from the BVM. Overall, I thought it's accurate, as the colour, improved heart rate and overall presentation match the monitor's interpretation. The end tidal carbon dioxide (ETCO2) is registering 18 to 22 mmHg, which is better than expected and with some fluid that should improve as well. The core temperature is 36.5 degrees Celsius, which is a little low but the blood sugar is 4.7 mmol/L, which is okay as well.

The paediatric Broselow tape is laid out beside the infant already. The weight is calculated and the proper epinephrine dosage is being drawn up while Lisa got a 24-gauge Intravenous (IV) catheter inserted into the infant's hand on her first attempt. We now have a fluid pathway right to the little person's heart. We can save a life more easily with any IV access so we are always thankful for anything and a bigger size is actually optimal if at all possible but any IV is a good IV in any sick or injured child. The bigger the angiocath, the better the IV will flow fluid but ideally a 24 or a 22 gauge is excellent. Just know that any IV is a good IV to my way of thinking.

The Arrow® EZ-IO® intraosseous vascular access system is available, but intraosseous access can take a few seconds. If we could obtain an IV line immediately it was not needed. If needed we can drill into any long bone or the lower leg to allow the administration of IV fluids and most emergency medications. I thanked Lisa, as she is a rock star, and inserted the IV successfully, ensuring it flowed well. I decided to initiate an IV bolus right away. I started to administer a 20-mL/kg bolus, as it's looking more like a trauma-related call. In no time, the CO2 was up to twenty-three which is also a great sign of better perfusion. The team is making the right decisions and today we have a hopeful outcome. Even if we are still doing CPR, it's a positive start in saving a life. Oxygen, IV therapy and a cardiac monitor are the essentials on every sick or injured patient as well.

The next plan of attack is medication administration and the only drug we can use in kids who are in real trouble while doing CPR is limited to just one drug today. The epinephrine is prepared and administered as per the standard PALS protocols using the Pediatric Broselow tape suggested dose and volume. I double-check the dose with another member just to make sure we don't make a lethal or sub-therapeutic dosage. Any significant medication mistake can mean our outcomes are less likely to succeed. So, it is worth double checking all dosages even when we are experienced.

Suddenly we could see the heart rate start to climb right away which is a great sign post-medication administration. It could be from the good ventilations, the effects of the oxygen on the hypoxic heart, the epinephrine, or it could be from the lifesaving fluids. Regardless, I was feeling more hopeful as it's looking like a better outcome than expected. In no time, we have changed the destiny of a little person in critical condition to having a chance to live, despite a terrible home situation.

In about two minutes the heart rate is up towards 80 bpm and the CO_2 is climbing to over thirty-seven so we decided to pause the chest compressions and watch the vital signs closely for thirty seconds to one minute. Our other crew is helping to intubate already and Lisa is looking for a backup IV site. She finds a small one and gets a second IV inserted and running but it's still an IV site so we will take it. The first BP is low so I elected to keep the next fluid bolus running and wondered if a low dose epinephrine drip or infusion might be a good idea. I wasn't sure so we waited a few minutes. It's best to give the body time to rebuild its functions to the normal levels without us altering the systems in too many cases. Overall, I think we have everything done that needs to be done initially.

I did a quick head to toe examination and it confirmed what I suspected as a child-abuse or a neglect case but that will be for the police and social services to look after in the days to come. Our job is to find injury and stabilize the child while ensuring he is kept safe from additional harm. Our dispatcher updates us that the PICU is going to be airborne in about ten minutes with a pediatrician that STARS helicopter was picking up from the University Hospital – Stollery roof. A quick loading of the equipment and they will be in the air and coming in low and fast. In no time, our pediatric specialist would be landing to take over our little broken and sick child. The gifted pilots will ensure the crew is brought to us in the fastest and safest approach. They are the unrecognized heroes most days on our teams.

Thank God, the cavalry is coming faster than our guardian angel's can drive and they can do the transport in a much quicker, a safer style with the experts providing lifesaving care at all times. We elected to start a safe and slow transport to the local ER. They will perform the rest of the required care and the advanced care in the local hospital with the local emergency physician and the greatest nurses in my world. We all were kept very busy helping save the life of one little child and in no time, we are transporting carefully. One of the extra police officers offers to bring our second unit and follows us to the local ER.

We are required to keep the initial RCMP officer who performed CPR for us and he will ensure the evidence is maintained and documented carefully. This is to try to ensure the guilty parties are dealt with correctly and hopefully this never happens to any other child. The teamwork displayed today was amazing and as we left the scene I said a silent prayer and thanked God this call is getting better and not worse. After the call is over everyone will need a mental health break. We will have more than deserved a free coffee break.

On arrival at the local ER we are taken into a trauma room. The staff swarm us and they rapidly take over patient care. The hospital staff would also keep Ken, my ride-along, involved. Becca, Tana and Lynn who are just a few of the great staff of the ER staff happily kept Ken busy and showed him the roles of the ER staff while I went to write my ePCR. Looking back, our other crew is such a lifesaver and they also helped my partner get our unit back in order, as I was busy. I asked the ER doctor to show Ken all the extra stuff and introduced him as one of our future employees and made him part of the team; even if he's only a ride-along, he matters. Looking back at our other crew, they were the real lifesavers on this call. They had our back for the complete call.

After a call is done it's time to document it all at the right time and in the right order. Thankfully, we get our times from our computer aided dispatch (CAD) system as well as our LP-15 and it helps me to start writing the call up in the proper order. It takes me about five minutes to go over what just happened in my mind to be able to chart it correctly. I kept checking to make sure I had the right times and the correct order of the procedures. I'm thankful our LP-15 has the vitals and the times of the interventions for the most part because it makes our ePCR much more accurate. I want to be as exact as I can, especially since this is likely to end up in court over the next year or two.

As I'm sitting trying to get my thoughts in order, one of the ER nurses noticed me looking off into space and I'm sure she felt my pain. I got a quick hug as she knew my troubles by just looking at me. She is one of my favourite ER nurses and she knows how our days can be. Some days the bad calls suck the life out of us. She understands the repeated attacks to our mental and physical health as well as the pain we feel after this type of call. Another staff member grabs us all a coffee, which was a lifesaver for sure. I could then get back to the electronic patient care report (ePCR). Even if it was too hot, the coffee was what I needed to give me the liquid courage to face the rest of this call. It could always cool as I made my way through the electronic patient care report.

As soon as I was done the ePCR and ready to book back in service, the PICU staff was already in the room and taking over the care. The chest X-ray showed pulmonary contusions and the abdomen showed distention; the fast scan showed free fluid. I cursed at the circumstances that lets this happen to little children. The RCMP relay there is a history of crystal meth and fentanyl abuse with the parents. That makes me even angrier that they still have a child living in such a disgusting apartment that is not safe or clean enough to keep animals in. It seems so wrong. Sometimes our society has better rules on the care of animals than people.

Then I thought about this and other calls we were doing weekly and wondered why the hell we spend millions on Narcan® kits instead of Adrenalin kits for patients with anaphylaxis history. We hand the Narcan® kits out like candy but nobody gives a thought to about why the people are doing drugs in the first place. Maybe addressing that concern would solve so many problems but we are a BAND-AID® society so it's simply ignored. We look the other way. We support people killing others all for drug money. I just hope someday parents will need a license to be able to bring a kid home from the hospital and will need to prove they can look after a child to keep him/her. Home care should do home visits and schedule the post-natal visit after the birth to ensure the family is coping and the baby is safe not just once. In this case, something went terribly wrong. In this case, the system ignored the red flags and the problems and the child paid the ultimate price.

After about an hour the little one is flown away to an urban PICU and will have the most appropriate investigations and care. Most likely a computer tomography (CT) and additional X-rays will be needed to find all the broken pieces. In time, with the miracles of medicine and some expert care, his fate will be decided. Sadly, we might never know the outcome but as he's in the hands of the best people in the world, it's out of our hands. We were told to make our way to the local RCMP station as they are having an informal debriefing, which is a very therapeutic way to deal with this type of trauma.

The informal debriefing is a non-punitive, non-judgmental setting for everyone. We are free to talk and say our feeling or our thoughts about the events of the call. Even if we are unsure or are second-guessing ourselves about our care such as "did we make the right decisions" or "did we make mistakes" no one ever criticizes us. It's purely a sharing, learning and debriefing event and its beneficial most times to all rescuers. Not everyone feels safe sharing and they don't attend for personal reasons. Every debriefing I have attended we give praise for the good aspects and we learn how to change our care in the cases to come. They will come just as the sun will get up tomorrow despite our bad nights. It will happen even if we are not ready for it.

Over the years, I have noticed these informal debriefings after serious calls bring our EMS, fire and police services even closer together and it helps to form one big family. There are times debriefings are not needed but sometimes it's a really good way to share stories and to lessen a person's stress. It's good to know we are never alone after a bad event. It's good to see others care and it's okay to be affected by the terrible events we endure at work. The longer you're in the EMS industry the more you realize we need to work as one.

Sadly, the incidence of PTSD may not be decreased with critical incident stress management (CISM) sessions. I agree we need them but there is a right time and a right place to perform a CISM session. Informal sessions in the past have done us more good than the formal sessions and I have never understood why. I think the problem we all missed out on was that CISM was never meant to be therapy. They are not the same. Some problems need one-on-one intervention with someone you trust and someone that can never come back at you. I would strongly suggest not using an employer or anyone in a supervisory role.

Sometimes the best therapy is with a small group of people that were there at the event and who are from the same service. Interagency CISM is a start but only a small part of the big picture in healing. Just know sometimes people with the best intentions can actually cause PTSD to be worse through the use of CISM or formal debriefing. The more we are involved and the closer we are to the events, the more impact we will feel despite being supported after the fact or after the event. The take-home message I got was crystal clear to ensure we always looked after our people before, during and after the emergency events.

Looking back over the last several years, we have seen and lost EMS family members from suicide due to PTSD. We are also losing people to compassion fatigue and also through them giving until they have nothing left to give. Sadly, we will likely lose many more to alcoholism and accidental or intentional overdose from illegal or prescription medications. Once we start down the wrong road, trying to cope with stress or by looking after stress the wrong way, it becomes unhealthy for many practitioners. Even with a backup system, people fall between the cracks of life. The "terrible or bad calls" we will see in a year, let alone a lifetime, are mind-blowing.

Today is one of the days that shows when we work as a team we make a difference. If it wasn't for the police on the scene as quickly as possible we would have been delayed entry and the child would have died. It could have been one of our local firefighter family members as first responders to this call who needed ALS care immediately. No matter the "what ifs" it was meant to work out the way it did. We came as a team and we intervened as a team. Thankfully the call transpired as it did with the members that were meant to be at the scene. Of all the things that could have gone wrong, the outcome was nothing short of a miracle despite the fact the little one was so injured. Thankfully the PICU staff is the experts in making this child survive the most terrible life imaginable.

Over two more cups of the best coffee in the world we needed to get back out, as another crew is currently covering us. We also knew that our night crew was called in early to cover us so we could attend the debriefing event so they are also part of the team. Thank God, our system has a brotherhood and a sisterhood of people that care. It wasn't always this way but thankfully it is now. With the coffee, I had enough energy to smile as my partner gave Ken and me a big group hug before getting back to work. Lisa smiles at me knowing the pain but she too will help me work it out over time. That is what team members do for each other and we were a team. Magically we were much more than a team for we performed miracles together despite the roadblocks we faced in life.

We booked back on and our night crew is off the hook for the next call. Medic-Five crew acknowledges that we are back in service and we thank them again for the extra help. We are free to go and fuel up and then we need some down time; as long as no calls come in we are okay to relax. In no time, we are back at base and we have only an hour left on our shift until it's over. The rest of the shift slowly goes past and with about fifteen minutes left, our relief is back on and smiling, they are more than willing and ready for the pending night shift. I was so happy to see them but still we had to visit for another ten minutes before we could get out the door and head home. I had Pebbles and Tinsel awaiting and ready to rumble.

We would take my trusty 1978 yellow F-250 and head east of town and find a spot for them to run like the wind. God, they loved that truck and everything it represented. Freedom and the fresh air blowing past was probably the most important but sitting beside me was the ultimate treat. My yellow truck and the pair of goldens were all part of my informal PTSD therapy session. Just by driving it and rolling down the window the wind at my side made the world just a little less bad. Pebbles and Tinsel would take turns riding next to me with mostly Tinsel having her head out the open passenger window enjoying one more day of freedom. They always smile and they never said not to any adventure 24/7.

My drive home was uneventful but something was still bothering me more than it would normally. I was thinking about why the little one got into this position or was placed in harm's way today and why the system never caught it. I vowed to call the administrator who is a friend of the Adult Children and Postnatal Care Program in the morning and ask the question that was left unanswered in my head. It should not happen but I needed to find out what our EMS service could do to prevent a similar disaster. Then I thought I should ask the ER doctor tomorrow about the outcome on this patient in PICU.

Tonight, will not be a good sleep. It won't be the first time I couldn't sleep after such a call. Sadly, I would soon realize it would not be the last. Tinsel never left my side all that long night. She knew I was hurting. Pebbles just simply guarded my door so I could sleep as much as possible.

The next day shift was slow and we only had one emergency call all morning. Ken spent most of the morning with Lisa going over our EMS equipment and protocols while I did my own thing. I got to chat with the on-call physician and the outcome looks promising for the little one. The RCMP member likely saved the little one's life by his quick actions. Starting CPR immediately and not thinking about it – he never even went to his car for a pocket mask or anything. He just made a decision and proceeded to try and save a life. That's what the EMS system is all about most days. Thankfully just the right trained police officer walked in and knew what to do. They sometimes simply ignore the personal protection hazards as they don't have a CPR mask handy or in their pocket so they just do mouth-to-mouth anyway which for kids simply saves lives.

Thinking about the call made me appreciate the good people in our world even more. Many people in similar circumstances do the same thing. Most don't think about the personal complications or concerns, they just do what they can with what they have and that's what truly saves lives. The next talk to the home care was not as promising and then I found the breakdown in the perfect world when the system misses the problems that should have been addressed or fixed. Not every system has a failsafe and this is why we can't prevent all disasters in a perfect world. We simply learn to react to a stimulus or respond to problem like it is the only thing to do.

Apparently, the Adult and Prenatal care group had a complaint lodged about the infant by a neighbour and nothing was done about it. Paperwork was filed in an office and never discussed again. It was our health care politics at its finest. They vowed to address it as a team and would be following up with the social services staff that also missed the opportunity to intervene. It was just another system fighting the cuts and recent reduction of staff due to funding issues. Health care cuts and interagency communication problems make everyone's day worse in certain circumstances. Perhaps someone's head will roll over this, but most likely not. Some issues just create more bureaucracy and solutions become just that more complex in the end. Hopefully next time the system works better for the sake of all kids that are out in harm's way.

I was just sitting thinking why they keep cutting essential services and wondering why we reward provincial health care administration with outrageous bonuses for saving money and then give some an extra $350,000 bonus for "risk pay." Someone should set fire to the whole system and rebuild it from the grassroots. I always thought health care and disease prevention should start at the patient level and work towards the hospital setting. Prevention of illness and disease should be the primary focus but it's not in our modern healthcare system. Someday the system may be accountable but I don't think it's happening anytime soon. The accountability is not present in a huge complex system where people are rewarded for our traditional sickness model. I was thinking about so many issues and realized our system was more mixed up than I knew.

Our next call was to the local baseball field for an injured child. We were almost at the end of our last day shift so it would be our last call. Thankfully Ken is still doing a ride-along and will see one more interesting call with our unit. The dispatch information was a suspected fractured leg of a young girl running in the outfield. We were en route and heading about two blocks towards the location of the injured patient but our siren wasn't working and our emergency lights were not flashing. Then at the same time we both started to laugh, as it's a rookie mistake – I realize I had forgotten to turn on the master power switch. Without that, nothing in the patient compartment or the emergency equipment works. One simple click of the master power switch to the "On" position and the lights and siren are finally working. Now people are moving out of our way. Whoops! It's a little thing but still funny just the same to two old timers. We both needed a good laugh right about then anyway. Sometimes things happen to show we are human.

At least this should be a straightforward call for a change, as we both needed a non-stressful call. On arrival, we found our patient was a twelve-year-old female with a broken lower leg. She was running and her foot got caught in a hole, twisted and broke within seconds. The poor girl's leg looks nasty. The lower third is deformed and the ankle fractured, dislocated or both but only an X-ray will tell the real truth. Her friend is crying and holding her hand tight. She's crying and the coach is crying too. I was almost ready to cry too. But big guys don't cry or at least that's what they say. "Must be the damn dust in my eyes." In no time, we have the situation under control and everyone has a job. I grabbed her other hand and told her we have just the right medication to make her ankle pain go away. I told her it's okay to cry but I will make the pain go away very quickly. I also told her friends she will need her cast signed tomorrow and to bring a good marker when they came to see her at the hospital.

I get her name and she got my name right away. Her name is Amie. I introduced her to Lisa and Ken. Lisa and Ken walked up with our kits right behind me. I thought that Entonox was a good idea to start with until the real drugs were ready. I asked Ken to grab it from the side door of the unit and I knew it was time to start the IV, sedate her correctly, then straighten and splint the nasty fractured leg. We ensured the parents were called and they will meet us in the local ER. After the Entonox was working, we started the IV. Lisa got it in right away as I was drawing up my meds. Morphine 2.5 mg increments up to 10 mg and Versed 2.5 mg x 2 and it's time to do the hard job. I waited an extra minute after she looked sleepy to ensure the medications were working and at least she wouldn't remember yelling, I hoped, when we straightened the badly broken leg. It always seems painful or hard to straighten a mangled extremity even with the right pharmacology. This is one thing no one likes to do but it's the right thing to do for the patient. With the right medication and the right effort, it's not so hard to do and after seeing and helping the doctors perform it, it gets easier.

I grabbed the ankle and supported it as well as the big toe. Lisa held the leg and Ken held her hand. We switched her to oxygen just to be safe as after the medications she might be a little too sedated, but for a good reason. It's a team effort and in seconds it's straight and there's only a slight cry, but that's allowed. We splinted it in a good normal or in as normal position as it will go for right now. The colour, the motor and the sensation were okay but it's not going to be great, due to the significant injury. I knew orthopedics would have a solution, but that is way above my pay grade. All we could do was simple basic care until they could fix it currently in a hospital setting.

We grabbed a scoop to get her off the ground easily and package her then off to the unit. In no time, she is on the monitor and we are off to the local hospital. We had the four lead cables on her and checked her oxygen saturations for the complete transport. Our ETC02 detector tells us she's still breathing normally although we would have expected the numbers to drop as she was hyperventilating a little bit on our arrival. I'm just worried and want to make sure her respiration and oxygen saturation were always kept within the normal range. During a sedation procedure, any patient can suddenly slow their breathing rate or have a lower tidal volume after the adrenalin is shut off because they relax too much. Even a simple fracture call can be a nightmare if we are not careful.

It's best to be prepared for the worst and expect trouble early in the call. In no time, she is waking up and talking more. I was smiling now as she was the one joking with me about how she gets a real cast now. Then she asked if she could get a pink cast, as that would be very cool and I promised to ask the ER staff the same question. I'd even pay the extra cost if needed but we would make it happen.

Apparently, my sedation selection was just enough. On arrival, the ER staff have a room ready for us with a set of worried and crying parents. The ER staff get us in the room and I give a quick report. The ER doctor has a little visit and looks at our handiwork and is happy. The hospital staff wheels her for a quick X-ray. I decided to wait and review the X-rays with Lisa and Ken because it was an excellent teaching opportunity. As soon as she's back, it's confirmed as a fracture. Our straightening was almost good enough but the ER doctor is going to adjust it a little more, apply a half slab and then call orthopedics in the city. All in all, it's a good job. We headed back to base to restock. Thankfully the outcome was okay as this is a scary injury for many, but kids will get quick attention and heal fast.

Our shift is almost over and the last two days have been eventful. We had time to sit and talk to my partner with Ken back at the base. Ken was fortunate to get such a good in-service and ride-along. Ken is one person that needs to come into our EMS family. Over the years, we know that when people show they are kind, they will be good in our profession. We both pushed Ken to get registered in the next EMR class and make sure he's working on how to get into the EMT class next. Heck, it's now the primary care paramedic (PCP) course but in my mind, it will always be the EMT class.

At the end of the day I took Pebbles and Tinsel for a five-kilometre walk and Tinsel made me throw the same stick about twenty times. Pebbles just walked ahead of me or right beside me and seemed closer than normal tonight. I can tell she feels my pain and she knows my day has been extra tough. I was just walking and listening to my iPod and a song came up that tells it all too well in my current situation. The song is by a great Canadian musician, "Bold and Beaten" by Matt Anderson. The words hit me like a rock right in the middle of my chest. The song was meant for me to hear that night.

As I stray out on my own
Become a stranger to myself
Walk away from all I own
Put my life onto a Shelf

I'm alone, but I'm not lonely
I've got friends everywhere I go
I've got a house, but still no home
I take shelter in my songs

I've been bold and I've been beaten
I've come ahead and I've lost
Everything I've been given
Has been worth the pain it cost

There's a lie behind my smile
A truth that can't be told
It's a load that I can't share
So I carry that load on my own

I've been bold and I've been beaten
I've come ahead and I've lost
Everything I've been given
Has been worth the pain it cost.

I listened to the song three more times as I walked along and I knew it was so true about me and even more, the song was really me. Somehow this one song is me and no one but me tonight will feel the pain, no one else cares about my honest inner feelings that I can talk to as I'm just too proud to call for help. Somehow, I was just meant to assume the pain and carry on at any cost. The lines "I've come ahead and I've lost Everything I've been given" was me. I never thought about it before but I'd helped others all my life. My inside was empty, or perhaps I was just overcome with so much pain and suffering over the last few tours of work.

I wanted to fix the world or change others' destiny but tonight I was just doing my best to stay alive and hold it together enough to keep going. I realized I needed a long holiday sooner rather than later. I will find a safe place to recharge my soul. I wanted to be somewhere else so the pain and suffering could take a little holiday. I knew that it would work out. It always has done in the past. "It has to for my life isn't ready to be over yet" I thought to myself.

The song was too real to me but most of my friends would never be able to see it and I could not say a thing to them. That was just not me. I thought, "Matt Anderson, you must have been in EMS at one time" as the song just keeps playing over and over in my head. I guess maybe your mom was a nurse. I got this message sent to me as I walked into the darkness with no fear of harm. My loyal golden retrievers would keep me safe and even though it was in the middle of the dark field I could see where to place every step without any extra light. Tonight, I was as safe as anyone could be in the world.

As I walked, the song just kept coming up over and over in my mind. The part "I'm alone, but I'm not lonely, I've got friends everywhere I go, I've got a house, but still no home, I take shelter in my songs," says more than any book I had read in years. I was missing the right person to share my pain. I needed just the right person to share the hurt and suffering we see over and over. Somehow it had to be lessened without harming others in the process. If I could just find some way to vent my built-up pain then I could go forward and know I was doing the right thing. A PTSD counsellor would probably be a good place to start but I was not ready. Lately I'd been doing my best but it wasn't enough anymore. I trusted Lisa, but I knew she had her own pain, her own suffering and I wasn't about to remove her smile or happiness at any cost. I was not about to let her assume my pain as well. That would not be fair or something I could burden her with for she was to special in my eyes.

I needed to feel alive and know that what I was doing in my life still counted or mattered. No amount of alcohol or drugs could ever make up for the lonesome heart or a heart full of personal pain. Someday I would find that someone to fix that void. Someone I trusted to share my worst secrets. I could not trust people that I knew and I never wanted people to think I was weak but then again, they knew I cared for everyone without question. I stood and prayed that someday it would happen when it was meant to, but regardless, I had to carry on. I knew life worked out the way it was always meant to. Until that day all I could do was to keep walking forward. I could not turn around now. Looking back doesn't fix the problems – it makes them harder to face – so I just kept walking along as a lost soul.

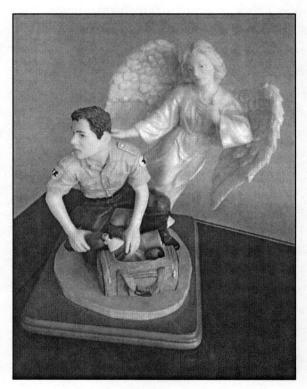

"Our Guardian Angel Works 24/7"

Chapter 4: No Way Out
"Running out of Options"

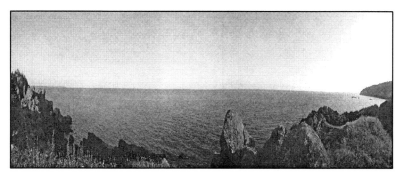

Running out of Options

I was having a good sleep in the recliner at the EMS base, silently waiting for a call but secretly hoping it never came. It was going to be a good tour as I was going on holidays in about fifteen more hours and I was already packed. I was heading back to Mosquito Creek, which is just north of Pared, Alberta for another planned much-needed mental health break. It was an amazing camping site with a busy little active creek running beside it that was surrounded by the mountains. I always tried to get the one camping spot that was furthest away from people. I would just sit and watch the water run past my feet for hours and nothing else in the world even mattered. I could feel the freshness of the fall air coming and it made me appreciate life more than most people would ever see, or feel in a lifetime.

I just had to make this last shift and one long night go away, then it was my time to drive away. I was partly packed and my Golden Retrievers would be in the truck and ready to head south to Red Deer and then west past Rocky Mountain House as soon as the morning sun made the horizon. It was so close I could almost reach out and feel the cold running water. Nothing ever happens just as we plan some days and I was about to find out my life and the many others in my EMS family would be changed forever.

The tones went off suddenly and I was up out of the chair and halfway to the door to get in the unit before I even knew it was a real call. We had just been dispatched to a single vehicle rollover about 10 km west of town. En route Lisa drove and I went through the motions to make sure we had the right location and that our backup unit was coming. I checked the computer-aided dispatch (CAD) on our unit's computer system a few times to make sure it was the right location. Our dispatcher confirmed one patient trapped and one person ejected and presumed dead on arrival (DOA). Being ejected at high speed is never a good sign and so often we know the outcome before our arrival. The local firefighters are coming with the rescue resources.

Thankfully the local volunteer firefighters have a few EMRs, an EMT and one paramedic on their volunteer roster so we had extra medical help if needed. Medic-Five lets us know they will be clear for backup in about two more minutes as they are just dropping off another patient in the local ER. They will not waste a second coming to our aid. They were the best of the best and I knew I needed them today more than most days. We had backup covered with the local RCMP and surrounding fire departments sending us all the support we could ever ask for so we had nothing else to think of but getting to the scene safely.

As we speed down the highway I thought our night is going to get real busy in about one more minute. I said a silent prayer and then

I put on my battle mask. War was already declared against the pain and suffering just around the next curve and we have lost one patient already. As we pulled up, the police (the local RCMP) have the scene controlled already. The fire rescue truck, a pumper and one other fire vehicle will be coming right behind us. They were all about two more minutes away. It was time for us to earn our pay and it would likely not be enough in the end if you considered the stress, risk of harm or even the possible threat of death all in the line of duty.

As we parked beside the police car that's blocking our scene in a good spot, we see the problem. One person looks to have been ejected after the truck hit an approach at high speed. The truck is lying on its side in about one foot of water. Lisa heads to the truck with a trauma bag and I grab the cardiac monitor and go to the ejected person lying about ten metres from the truck's bumper. As I walked up it was clear he was already dead on arrival (DOA). I checked for any signs of life but no pulses were present and there were no visible signs of any breathing attempts.

When he was ejected, something likely crushed the side of his face. His brain and head were most likely crushed or broken beyond repair. His left side was also broken and deformed and normally we would put the monitor on him but being he is dead and we have another patient, I just gave up on him and went to help Lisa. Sometimes destiny is not challenged. The second they hit the approach the vehicle was doomed and the crash become a fatal event for at least one occupant, the decision about living or dying is made by a higher power than us.

I wondered why he didn't have a seat belt on but when we see the open beer cans ejected around the accident scene, I had the answer to that really dumb question. I guess if people are drinking and driving, seat belts are most likely very optional and speed signs are only a suggestion. I know the legal system is so broken and that most of the drunk drivers get off or receive a lesser sentence; even when they kill people it doesn't seem to matter. I have hated lawyers and politicians for years for ignoring this ongoing problem.

We have more problems when they ignore the facts that we have more and more drunk drivers on our roads every year. The police work very hard to stop and charge the impaired drivers. But it seems the legal system fights to get them off on technicalities in almost every case. I swore to myself one more time as I found Lisa assessing the living patient lying in the truck still alive but beaten and very broken. I thought about the Matt Anderson song that keeps playing over and over in my head and I don't know why. *"I've been bold and I've been beaten, I've come ahead and I've lost, Everything I've been given has been worth the pain it cost."* was being played over and over in my mind for some reason. Somehow that song was meant to give me a message but for the life of me I had no clue what was coming in my near future.

Lisa yells over to me: "25-year-old male confused but seems to be stable otherwise." Lisa found multiple rib fractures with a flail segment to the left chest wall, a broken pelvis and a broken arm as well. "It also looks like he might have a closed head injury and is a little combative but not too bad" Lisa says to me. I had made my mind up already on the mechanism of injury as well as the combative behaviour that he needed a trauma center and STARS would be a great option for a rapid transport to the awaiting trauma team. "Do you need anything?" I ask. Lisa states, "Just a spine board and a cervical collar should be okay for now." I headed back to the unit and grabbed our spinal gear and the cervical collar kits along with our restraint straps. I also started thinking that he would need an advanced airway for transport but that thought could wait a few minutes.

Just then the fire units roll up and several members come to help us right away. The captain has a quick look and offers to roll the cab away to give us a much easier extrication. I was happy about that, as Lisa is looking after c-spine inside the truck for now and she looks to have it all under control. The fire crew throws a blanket over Lisa and the patient for now and we must wait for the roof to come off before extrication and patient stabilization could occur. The Jaws of Life is started and in no time our patient is going to be free. I decided to go back to the unit and spike a few normal saline (NS) IV bags as I wanted them ready as soon as the patient was free and in the unit.

Dispatch advises us that the STARS Air Ambulance is willing to fly if we want them and I acknowledge the request. They will be launched in a few minutes. They are most likely pulled out of the hangar with their engines started and warming up already right after we got our initial dispatch they would also be alerted of the serious call. After they do their warm-up and safety checks they will be airborne from the Edmonton International Airport (EIA) and heading towards us all while the pilots would be watching out for the conflicting inbound and outbound aircraft during their priority one launch. In several minutes, it will be STARS-3 to our rescue one more time. In almost every case it is the best mode of transport for the sickest patients.

Once STARS-3 are wheels up, they are climbing for altitude with every turn of the rotors providing the magic lift and they are up and away. As soon as they have the appropriate altitude they will turn their nose into the right direction and seek speed and altitude at the same time. Then they land in just the right spot and within thirty seconds, the crew is out and coming to help stabilize a very ill or very broken person. It was a well-oiled team that always tried to work to help alleviate pain, decrease suffering and prevent premature death. Lifesaving doesn't get much better than that.

We just updated the dispatcher that we will likely need to intubate him and he should be ready for flight on STARS-3's arrival if everything goes as planned. Before they land beside us in about fifteen minutes we will have two IVs in him running, his flail chest and broken pelvis will be stabilized. He will also be intubated correctly, and hopefully an oral gastric tube (or if they had no head injury we could insert a nasogastric (NG) tube) can be easily inserted to remove the excess gas from gastric distention. It will help remove the gastric contents, which is never a bad idea. Heck, we might even have time to insert a Foley catheter and then the trauma team will be extra happy to see the urine flowing into the catheter bag.

We could be a mobile intensive care unit for a few minutes. Anything we can do to help speed up the process to get the patient to the CT scanner in the city hospital is always a good idea. A "Pan Scan" as well as review by the trauma team is in order on arrival and the sooner the better for the patient's sake. We do our best not to waste any precious seconds of the golden hour with our trauma care. With the golden hour, so much time is lost in the dispatch sequence, and then the time it takes to get to the scene, followed by the time spent stabilizing a patient. Time is also taken deciding the most appropriate mode of transport. All of that eats up the precious seconds and sixty minutes runs past faster than you would think when you get busy trying to save a life.

Time is so valuable but also so precious. It is always best to plan for a medivac decision sooner rather than later, as it's precious time used wisely. Many times, we would dispatch the helicopter based off of our dispatch information because it was just logical not to waste precious time. Simply from the mechanism of injury (MOI) you could already put them on standby and if you were lucky they would be almost ready to launch when they got the request for help.

As we were extricating the patient, I thought about how far the trauma care has come from when I started in EMS. We have learned to always start two IVs as big as possible unless there are unforeseen complications or the injuries are trivial. We love to use Ringer's Lactate in burns or later on in trauma care in certain cases but almost all protocols call for EMS to provide normal saline boluses if needed to maintain a stable BP or a mean arterial pressure (MAP) over 65 in most patients and we were expected to keep the MAP over 75 in the head-injury patients. Essentially, we need a good MAP to perfuse our body after major injury or with many complex medical conditions that cause hypotension which is low blood pressure (BP).

In most cases we will also want to administer Tranexamic acid (TXA) 1 gram IV over ten to twenty minutes if it's indicated in hypovolemic (excessive internal or external bleeding) trauma cases. Trauma care has improved greatly in North America in the last fifteen to twenty years; many lives have been saved with the use of modern Advanced Trauma Life Support (ATLS) care practices.

I got a little chuckle from the thought that today the NG will even help to remove the excess alcohol, excessive gastric distention and the stomach contents in this case. The patient paid good money for the alcohol and we try our best to take it back and dump it down the drain. Thankfully our crazy legal system can't charge us for taking his high away – unless it gets any dumber, which isn't unrealistic in our lifetime. Now that is a stupid thought. I must be really tired to think this crazy stuff up. "If lawyers had to work with us for a week during their education process maybe they would help fix the broken system" is what I was thinking just before we needed to intubate our patient.

Thankfully our scene is very controlled and we don't have to worry about our safety tonight. The extra fire department members and a few extra sheriffs are helping the police to set up a landing site right beside us for STARS. The highway is now closed off to everyone except emergency vehicles. Our backup unit is also en route and will give us additional help to intubate and package yet another fine, intoxicated citizen. I wondered why he was so lucky but his friend died and then my random thoughts were cancelled because it's time to get to work as the roof is off. After more than twenty years we still see drunk drivers and nothing makes them go away. They just keep driving and killing innocent people and nothing or nobody in power seems to care or make an effort to stop it.

Lisa was smiling to me as we helped to slide the patient out of the vehicle. The funny thing was that she just told me at the start of our shift tonight we would be busy and I told her we were going to sleep all night long. Then she said that tonight we would be intubating one more time before my holidays even got started. I told her with one courageous look this is all her fault as she jinxed us but she laughs even more at me. She knew exactly what I was thinking. Our weird sense of humour always helped us both relax even more and it gets us ready to save lives with so much less stress than there could be, as it calms us both down. When you were in a stressful situation a little appropriate laughter went a long way to help lessen the tension. It makes the team flow even better.

We are more than ten times as good providing patient care when we are a team. I looked at her one more time and I knew she was my real-life guardian angel. After this call we were going to have one long talk. I knew I could trust her and she would help me. I knew right then she could take my pain and turn my life around. I have finally found my miracle to help solve my lifetime accumulation of work related stress. Somehow, I knew she would be able to reach my broken spirit and help me heal from the inside. We all need someone we can share our pain with and a life time in EMS can create some pretty bad memories.

As we place the patient in the unit he's still very combative. We are not sure if this is a case of acute alcohol poisoning or a closed head injury. The patient has no obvious signs of a bad head injury but as soon as we start to cut the clothing off we will know more. The backup crew arrives and we have Bridget and Peter ready to help out. Peter is the newest paramedic and Bridget is one of the senior EMTs with our service and a mother of three kids. I think she has been an EMT for about fifteen years so she will keep Peter out of trouble. Bridget is the real boss and Peter keeps Bridget happy by doing the right stuff on every call – they get along just like an old married couple. It is so cute to watch them talk back and forth. I am a little intimidated sometimes trying to be her boss, as she would tell me in a no-nonsense way what we needed to do. I guess that was the super-mom coming out and it was appreciated in many ways.

Tonight, everyone has a job assigned and I'm the ringmaster when it comes to documenting this on the ePCR for this event but everyone knows this call is Lisa's all the way. Peter will intubate and Bridget is helping to draw up the rapid sequence induction (RSI) medications. With the help of some good pharmacology he will be ready to be intubated safely and have a magic GCS of 3/15 from some great IV-induced chemicals. Lisa is starting the IV's and as soon as they are ready we can start to get the airway secured.

The high flow nasal prongs are on at 15-LPM already and pre-oxygenation is looked after. I started my quick head-to-toe and I exposed the chest and abdomen to see the mark of the steering wheel onto his chest and I agreed with Lisa, it could be a flail segment. So at least we know he was the driver even if the police can't or won't ever be able to charge him and get a conviction. If he lives, they might get a charge of manslaughter but normally it doesn't make it to court in all too many cases. Ironically it will just be another drunk driver and he will live to drink and drive again unless he somehow figures a way out of his careless lifestyle. Sometimes the system just sucks. I'm not saying anyone is to blame but I was just thinking the system is pathetic to not try and stop this tragic outcome before it gets this far. If you added it up we have killed thousands every year across Canada and around the world every year and somehow it never makes the world news.

I will never know why the driver was the lucky one and the passenger was not. It never fails to surprise me that the drunks seem to survive more often in accidents with the passengers often becoming the fatalities. This makes no logical sense unless they are so drunk they just bounce like a rag doll. Strangely we can come onto a scene and have three people dead and then we come across the drunk driver who is still alive. It doesn't seem right but it happens all too often. Sometimes we just don't have the answers to such deep questions. Then when the police end up the case with no charges pending due to our great justice system, it makes me sick.

I ask this question over and over "How many people have to die?" for us to get our shit together and say enough is enough. One of my police friends stated only about ten percent of all cases get a conviction. Many cases are plea-bargained away and only a few get what they deserve for the crime. In the olden days, it was simple – if you did the crime you do the time. Today you can get away with murder or driving drunk and chances are you never do any jail time.

As the thoughts of the drunk driver situation occurred one more time in my mind at light speed I completed the exam and I noticed the pelvis or the left femur is shorter than the right and slightly rotated outwards with his leg rotated as well, just a little further than the normal position should allow. I suspected a femur dislocation or a fracture at the neck of the femur. We quickly pulled on the big toe on the left leg to get the ankles to the same length and then bound the ankles together with a figure eight. Just to be safe we bound the pelvis as well but I'm sure it's not the pelvis. Either way no one will be mad at us for trying our best. I could see the leg move back to the right location and the pulses and colour are still good so I'm happy with that for now; with a little traction applied it looked better.

A quick summary is closed head injury most likely with a possible flail chest and pulmonary contusions highly expected, a possible pelvic injury and left femur fracture or dislocation. It is somewhat better than the dead guy so it could have been much worse.

The LP-15 is on and his pulse rate is about 120 bpm with no ST changes on the monitor but I delegated a 12-lead just because of a possible cardiac contusion. We know it's not easy to see the subtle electrical changes in the cardiac contusion cases but we looked anyway. Our Sp02 is 100% which we expected and the ETC02 is also in the safe range around forty-five via the nasal prong C02 sampler so it's slightly high but our intubation will fix that with some extra ventilations in no time. The core temperature is 36.4° Celsius which is a little too cool for trauma patients but okay for isolated head injuries, in theory anyway. We will try to keep him from getting any colder to prevent increased complications.

When we considered his suspected injury, I thought about what they taught us in ensuring the brain stayed at a normal temperature. The trauma lecturer talked about how the brain was so delicate that it was similar to a delicate fruit or vegetable. "The brain must be protected" was the golden rule. The rule actually was about warming up the brain in injury or illness conditions. Just think "the warmer the vegetable the faster it rots" which was something I learned many years ago at a Critical Care Conference in 1986 and never forgot it. Well today his brain temperature was okay but the oxygenation and cerebral perfusion had to be optimal and the ETC02 needed to be maintained at a unique balance.

Ultimately the best way to ensure the brain was protected was to intubate him for transport. As the patient was already altered in his mentation, it could be easier than normal to get him safely intubated. We know it will take less pharmacology to induce a good chemical sedation to enable us to intubate him freely but might take more to keep him from waking up due to the effects of alcohol.

Our IVs are running and we elected to give a fluid bolus and think TXA 1 gram over twenty minutes was a good idea. This patient has signs of internal injury. With active bleeding, the use of TXA is part of our trauma protocol. Someone was grabbing the 1-gram vial and had added it to the mini bag. It was running in no time. The BP is a little lower than we would expect at 94/52, which could be from decompensated shock but also partly from a cervical spine injury. It's not a clear case of neurogenic shock but could have some potential as the heart rate is compensating so well. With the fluid bolus, the BP should come up and may help decrease the tachycardia (fast heart rate) over time. If it doesn't, then we know the bleeding might be worse than expected. It was too bad we didn't have a Fast Scan but STARS-3 does and they can scan him on their arrival if they want, or inflight. They also have blood products available if needed and that might be an option. It would be used after a few IV boluses are given and the tachycardia persists if we suspected a lower than expected hemoglobin (Hgb).

I started to think about the changes over the years in how we treated our trauma victims. We have gone away from using Trauma IV tubing that could give massive IV boluses of IV fluid or blood products in minutes. More recently we've moved to the passive IV use in hypovolemia therapy, which is proving that limited volumes of fluid in uncontrolled bleeding conditions might help patients get to the operating room (OR). We learned our lesson in the Vietnam War by just giving blood or cold blood products puts people in shock and that was not always a good idea. By giving them some isotonic fluid first whether it's normal saline (NS) or Ringer's Lactate (RL) also known as Hartman's Formula was a good start. Now that we are using TXA with our bleeding patients we can save many more lives. I just wish we could get the mast pants back and it would be a perfect world. Someday it will come back but likely after I retire, I am afraid. But it will happen, you can mark my words.

We elected to administer Midazolam 2.5 mg and Fentanyl 100 mcg IV, then added Anectine® (Succinylcholine Chloride) 120 mg IV because this person was about 85 kg and anything around 1.5 mg/kg is a good dose to start with. Our crew was ready with the bougie and the video laryngoscope if we needed it. We have the

King Vision® as a great backup if needed and it gets used more often than it should. Since the introduction of the (Gun Elastic) bougie, our intubation rates have increased to over 95% which is better than most services. In the first attempt, we passed the 7.5 cuffed endotracheal tube (ET) past the vocal chords, the cuff was inflated and we have a positive end tidal wave from with a reading of 38 mmHg which is okay for a start. We increased our ventilation rate a little faster to get the ETC02 to around 32 to 35 mmHg as this person is most likely a closed head injury.

The oral gastric tube was inserted and our ET tube was secured with the Thomas Tube clamp and was set at 22 centimeters right at the teeth. Our airway is secure and we just need to monitor the Sp02 and ETC02 to ensure nothing goes wrong. The ventilations were easy and there were no problems noted at the present time so we all can breathe a little easier as well. Today our pharmacology worked just like it was supposed to when all worked right.

We then noticed the heart rate had dropped to around 100 bpm which tells us the IV fluid is likely helpful. On our secondary exam, we noticed battle signs starting which made us more confident that this is likely a fairly good closed head injury. Normally battle signs can take up to six hours to develop or be visible in milder head injury cases. Once we see this cardinal sign we know it's likely a significant head injury patient. Our repeat chest examination also has multiple flail signs on palpation. We can easily feel multiple broken ribs, which is scary as most times we suspect it but it's not confirmed without X-ray and CTs.

As we are ventilating at the correct rate and with non-excessive pressures already it's going to be okay but we have to be careful not to increase the ventilation pressure too much and make a tension pneumothorax occur. Unless we blow a pneumothorax, the lungs should keep ventilating – even being bruised and filling with some blood in the most damaged areas they will still work, just not as well. I wondered if we already had a small pneumothorax, but a hemothorax (bleeding in the lung area) is more likely today even without seeing the subcutaneous emphysema yet.

The abdomen was unchanged and the pelvis was secured tightly with our straps. The left leg was unchanged with good colour and pulses still present. I was very glad to hear the familiar sound of the STARS-3 helicopter coming overhead. That is one part that never gets boring to see the helicopter coming in fast, complete a circle and make a controlled safe approach. They were just doing the circle to get lined up for the perfect approach. The pilots would look for unseen hazards from the air on every approach. Overall, this call has gone well except for the fact there was one-person dead; it's going to turn out better than it might have. Today we will at least save one person which is a very good start.

Thankfully today these two only have hurt themselves and didn't take out an unexpecting family on the highway or even worse, hit a school bus with kids so it's much better than it could have been. In another minute, our vital signs are repeated and our patient is stable and ready for flight minus the Foley catheter, which we never got in, but it's not a big deal today. In less than a minute the flight crew is hopping into our unit and taking over the patient care in record time. They have another flight pending so they will get going to try to clear up as soon as possible. Today it's going to be grabbing a patient and leave in record time. Lives are on the line and the aircrew are making our job extra easy, as now we have no transfer to do, which is a good way to end a serious call.

STARS-3 has an inter-hospital transfer they have been requested to assist in, as the hospital needs a flight physician to help out so they do their best to accommodate the patient care that is needed by a small rural hospital when it is needed. If they are delayed the patient will receive an alternate form of transport which may not be the best, but that's part of a normal day. We all try to do our best.

Thinking back, the time when we used them most often was three rapid back to back flights and in total they transported six patients all from one bad accident, which is nothing short of a miracle of air transport.

The transfer of care goes easily and in no time the patient is secured in STARS-3 and they are getting ready for an almost immediate take off. Today they never even shut the helicopter down and it was a hot load, which means the rotors keep running. Our job is done but our unit is a huge mess and we will be out of service until we are restocked and cleaned up. We thanked everyone and I asked Lisa to drive so I could get the ePCR done on the way to town. Just before we left the scene I gave her a big high five and said, "Lisa you are an angel." She just looked right at me and smiled and gave me a magical wink. I had never seen that look before and it made me feel very special inside.

En route to town I was writing the ePCR and didn't see the semi-truck cross the centre line and come right at us. Lisa yelled, "Hang on!" as she swerved hard to the right ditch but it was already too late. The semi was destined to hit our unit and Lisa gave me my life by letting the semi nail her side of the unit. Both vehicles hit at 100 km. The impact was like 200 km against a solid brick wall. The ambulance couldn't take the impact. The airbags and seat belts helped out but not enough for Lisa. I never even felt the impact as my world just went blank. It's like we were falling but never touched the ground. I heard the tires screaming for traction, then the sound of metal bending or breaking and glass breaking but I didn't feel anything. I could smell the blood and I could taste it but I didn't see the crash. The whole accident happened so fast it could not be measured.

I never got to see our backup crew trying to save Lisa along with the STARS-2 crew that was diverted to our crash site. I don't remember who was even intubating me right after the crash but I heard afterwards it was the volunteer fire paramedic who is a close friend. Everyone helped from the local RCMP to the local fire rescue teams that were packaging me for a rapid flight to the trauma centre. I didn't get to see the team work so hard to save Lisa but she truly was an angel because after the impact she was already gone. In seconds, I bet she was looking at me from above and holding onto me for dear life and would not let me die. I just kept flying through the air for what seemed forever. I couldn't remember how long as I felt a sensation of flying in the midst of clouds.

I completely missed my volunteer fire department friends cutting me out of the passenger side with a mangled vehicle chassis that seemed to melt all around me, but I was intact. It was a very painful job for my friends. They worked as a meticulous team along with the other local surrounding volunteer Fire Department crews coming to help as well. They had two rescue teams working at one time. There was never a power struggle – it was just one team of rescuers doing their best.

It was likely the most difficult, challenging and painful extractions from the mangled mess they had ever had to do to get me out. Then they had to free Lisa. I missed our friends crying and working as a team even with tears running along with their sweat but they never quit. They made extra sure they never hurt her and they carried her with love to the waiting ambulance with an honour guard ensuring she was protected from harm. The same people used the police vehicles and fire crews with the extra fire trucks to escort her to the local ER where she was cared for with more tears and love as they prepared her to go to the provincial coroner's office as required by law.

Not one person had dry eyes including the older most hardened physician that took time to sit with the staff, and he too cried with them. Many didn't know that Lisa was my guardian angel in the STARS-2 helicopter and they missed the part that I was unstable and she was busy keeping me alive with her spirit at my side. I'm sure that day was the one-day that everyone worked without complaint and didn't quit until there was no one else to help.

I was completely oblivious that our unit was totally destroyed by the impact of the semi and the rescue tools were making it a tin can with no recognizable shape left. Somehow, I should be thankful that our air bags deployed and I had my bulletproof vest on. That most likely saved my chest and vital organs from injury. The seat belt most likely helped to save my life; even if it didn't save Lisa, it saved me. I still should have died but somehow, I was spared. My guardian angel I actually knew before we left the last accident. That Lisa was my guardian angel all the time but I didn't realize until just before the crash. I should have seen it but I never did, until it was almost too late. I knew the second she gave me that once in a lifetime magical wink who she really was in my mind.

I missed the huge memorial service for Lisa the following week as I was in a medically induced coma. It was the biggest memorial service performed for any EMS worker in the province held at the Civic Centre to accommodate the massive number of mourners. I missed my holiday because my plans had been changed in a heart-beat. My life was also changed forever. One person's lack of attention killed my best friend and almost killed me. I guess his punishment was fitting, but not the pain it cost his family for the many years to come. Some pain is not measurable. Grief can eat away a person's soul. My life was the only one spared and that makes me feel even worse than one could imagine. Why did she let me live and why did she need to die? It was my turn as I was the broken person.

I slowly woke up about a week later in an ICU and was extubated, still in a drug-induced haze. I could feel my body was broken but still part of me. My left arm and my left leg were still in a full cast. I had surgery to repair multiple fractures and then was put in an induced sleep to let my brain swelling go down. They knew that rest was the best thing possible. Slowly my secondary injuries resolved and my body systems went back to a steady state.

After some time, I started to notice the people around me but strangely many that I didn't know or I couldn't recall right away. My brain was foggy. Slowly my friends came in and showed me support and kindness as soon as they were allowed past the nurse's desk. In a few days, my central lines were out and I was back to being awake more than I was asleep.

The biggest question I had but just could not ask was "Where is Lisa?" Why was she not at my side? She wasn't one to ever miss out keeping me cheered up or to ignore my pain. Lisa had always felt my pain even if I never said a thing she knew my pain and would help me get through a bad day. I was terrified to ask and I knew it was bad but I could not bring myself to ask that question. I wondered how I could sneak out and go to her place and make sure she was okay. I wasn't sure where my keys were or where my truck was but I needed to go and find her. We had been on a call and my truck was already packed for my holiday but I don't remember ever going.

Why did I not remember my trip? It would have been my annual recharge trip and my puppies would be sitting beside the truck waiting to leave. They always knew when we packed that they were part of the travel team. Why were they not with me? They always slept in my room or beside me. Pebbles would guard the entrance to my door and Tinsel would curl up beside me to listen to my heartbeat. Why were they not with me? I wondered, but I could not bring myself to ask for I was to be scared for the real answer.

A day later they moved me to a private room and my EMS friends were waiting for me with my golden retrievers. They immediately jumped on my bed and refused to yield. Then I started to cry for the first time. They snuggled as close as possible and they would not move not even for the nurses caring for me. The nurses just worked around them and Tinsel watched their every move as Pebbles just lay beside me, closed her eyes and rested. It's then they slowly told me what had happened in the accident and what had happened to Lisa. I knew it was bad but this was way past anything I thought possible. Tinsel's heart simply matched mine and my pain slowly ebbed away.

I knew a few days back something was wrong as Lisa was not at my side and I knew something very bad must have happened or she would be there making me smile and we would laugh together. Pebbles and Tinsel just crawled tighter to me over the next several hours as my friends broke the news to me and slowly I understood pain that I had never known. I had one person in the world that believed in me. I had one person who had given me a reason to live and just like that, she was gone. I must have cried myself to sleep, for I could not stop crying.

Nothing could have taken away the pain and the deep loss I felt right then. Over the next few hours my friends just stayed and when I slept they still stayed at my side and waited for me to come back from my terrible dream. It had to be a dream. More likely it was just another nightmare. But this nightmare was different. It was much more painful.

When I woke up I had my loyal golden retrievers holding me tightly in bed and my friends were holding onto me and ensuring I was not going to be alone. They were now my sole protectors. They would and had looked after me for years and they had also saved my life when I should have died but somehow and for some reason, I was always spared. One of the nurses gave me some really good medications and I slowly faded onto a waiting cloud. My pain was gone for a little while before it was back. I was able to feel warm and loved by my friends even if I was still broken. I was now able to think a little better with less pain at least for a bit. It seemed in life I had pain everywhere all at the same time but I think the pain proved to me I was still alive.

The pain was never gone but for a few hours they had given me something that took the edge off it and it sort of made me completely numb and I lost track of time. My friend Leanne from the local hospital had not left my side for a long time. My kids finally took the puppy's home even when they tried to stay. In the end, I had to tell them nicely it was okay to go with the kids as they licked my face one more time and were off to get a Timmy's treat on the way home. They loved their cheese tea biscuits but would settle for the plain Timbits in an emergency. I knew they would be back again in the morning and they would again be at my side for as long as possible in another twelve hours.

The room was so silent with only the sound of the monitors audible. For hours, I never said anything and we just held onto each other. Slowly I started sharing the memories with Leanne about Lisa and then I realized by some magical way her spirit was still alive and she was in the room beside me. I could feel her presence. I could smell her perfume but more importantly, I could feel the presence of her heart. She simply told me as plain as day to let her go and in the next breath she said, "Get up and you fight this, damn you." That would be Lisa's exact words and after that moment I felt a peace come over me that I hadn't felt before.

I was never very good about going to church but I was spiritual and I believed in Christianity. I knew there was a heaven and I knew for sure there was a hell, but I wondered if it was most likely here on earth. Just knowing heaven was within reach was my "ace in the deck of cards" that life had dealt me. It was not visible to me, but it was not far away. It would have to wait as my job wasn't done yet. Even if I was broken, I knew somehow, I would get back to my EMS job. It would be a long painful trip but it was possible. I would do it for Lisa. Lisa would be at my side and she would assume the pain I could not handle.

Once I figured out I was meant to live my pain was less and my heart was suddenly at peace. For some reason, this tragic event was meant to be and my faith in keeping Lisa's spirit alive would not be wasted. My heart was still broken but the pieces were in my reach. If Lisa was my new guardian angel she would help put the pieces back together, then I would be able to fight this tragedy. I would go on. I knew I'd make it back to my EMS job. I would find a partner that could make it work. The management would need to find someone special that could put up with my unique ways. I knew I was alive for a reason and nothing was going to change my fight to make it back to work. As long as I could make it off this bed, I would crawl to the unit or I'd simply die trying. I was not afraid of dying but some days I was more scared of living.

Later on, in the evening I had some of my physician and nursing friends come to visit. One of my best friends was one of the staff trauma surgeons come to visit. He spent an hour with me and took his time. He made me feel that my purpose in life was to keep going. He also said that the hospital and STARS had set up a memorial fund for future EMS students as that was Lisa's wish. It would be her legacy to keep helping others even from heaven.

Then he looked into my eyes and touched my heart as he said my road to recovery was going to be slow but I would be back to work in six to twelve months. Spiritually, mentally and emotionally it was not as clear. There will be many personal inner challenges to meet and get over before that was ever going to happen. But he looked at me and said "if you want it, you will make it back up. You have been knocked down, broken but you're not dead for a reason. This world is not done with you yet. You are the only one that can fight this battle but we will be at your side every step of the way." He gave me a big hug and when he walked out he stopped at the door and looked back at me as he said, "Lisa still has your back, my friend" and just like that, he was gone. He was another one of my guardian angels and he was meant to be looking over me for all the right reasons.

I slowly thought about what he just said and I knew I was not as young as I once was, so I would not heal as fast as I would have in the past. I know the arthritis that will come along soon will remind me of the weather changes, especially on our cold winter nights. If everything healed, as it should, there was nothing to keep me from working when the time was right. I just had to find the courage and the willpower to make it happen.

I thought about the pain ahead and in some strange way I welcomed it. I knew as long as I could feel pain I was still alive. Sometimes it was the pain that made me want to fight to live. Pain was my friend. At least it was a start and I needed something to get me back up. I noticed the sound of silence more now than I had in the past. I just wanted the last several weeks to just go away or somehow not ever happen but that was not going to happen. I looked up towards the heavens and said, "Thank you God for my life but please look after Lisa." Then I slowly closed my eyes and held onto the belief that my life had a purpose as I fell back to sleep.

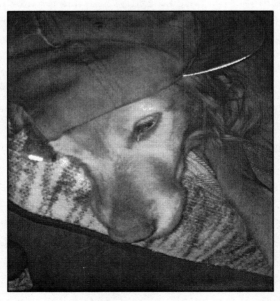

"Surviving a very bad day"

Chapter 5: Coming Back - Facing the Past

"Fixing the Cracks"

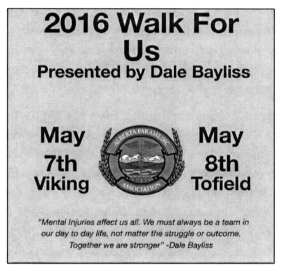

"No One Walks Alone"

The day came when I was ready to go back to work. I had been off for about seven months. The physiotherapist had pushed me when I was not willing to go on to the next day. She challenged me to get better and do enough to make myself stronger every day. Slowly she made me the person I used to be, but I was not the same. I would never be the same person. At the end of the day I knew I had no other choice but to keep walking ahead. A few times I would wake up and be terrified but I got the light on and saw that Pebbles and

Tinsel were still at my side. In the background, my music never stopped playing. I was still alive and that was all that mattered. I had people that believed in me and that had to count for something.

Music was my saving grace. It was what brought me some inner peace even if most people could not hear the message or take the time to appreciate the messages I got from the songs. I had many favourite songs that I just played over and over. They gave me inner strength and opened my heart back up to being in a better place. I could feel the pain worsen on some days, feel the suffering and know it was real. In some strange way, all the bad was pulled to the surface and slowly taken away. The music had a way to my soul and it was my therapy for the bad times in the past. It took the fatigue from my thoughts and made it into light.

One day I knew I was ready to go back to work physically but mentally and spiritually I was still broken. I would not be ready unless they found me a partner who could spend the time to help me get back on my own two feet. One night I went for a long walk and after about ten kilometres I stopped and prayed for some peace. I prayed for God to look after Lisa as I often felt her presence but could never see her. I asked God to send me someone to make my days better and on my way home I knew something had changed in me. It was like a thousand pounds had been lifted off me.

On the drive into work I was having palpitations. I had left fifteen minutes early and it was lucky I did because I had to pull over and calm down before I could finish the short drive to work. I just knew I had to go on and today would be a hard day. When I pulled into the parking lot I was okay and as I walked into the side door of the office I was greeted by Sarah. She gave me a really long and sincere hug and we both cried for a minute. Sarah said she had a new job today and I said "Great" for I knew she would be an excellent EMT. Then she looked into my eyes and I cried as she told me she was going to be my new partner and my own personal training officer. I could not have not have found a better partner to get me back to my old job. I cried as I hugged her one more time. I knew my prayers had been answered. There was no way I could come back with the wrong person. One of us would end up gone for good and it would have to be me. Today I was given a second chance in more ways than I would ever know.

Once I knew I was assigned to partner with Sarah, who was one of my strongest past EMT student. With her help, I could start to relax and breath so much easier knowing I had a fighting chance to make it back to who I needed to be as a paramedic. Somehow, someone in management knew that even though she was a new EMT graduate, she would be the perfect partner for me. That would be Kenn and Greg on my side for they knew me and they were someone I could and would trust with my life and knew she would be the right person for our team to work. When we had her as a student with Lisa we took turns quizzing her and mentoring her, even on the ALS skills.

We always had a good rule and it would hold for a lifetime. We had taught Sarah from her first call that we had each other's back and what happened on our shift was dealt with by the team. We never left a tour without resolving a difficult problem. We broke the problems apart and found a solution. Even if it was painful or hard on someone, it always was resolved. Sarah would follow the tradition Lisa and I had perfected.

In the past, it didn't matter if Lisa was attending or I was for we always made the students come together as one of the team. They were going to be mentored, not dictated to, while on my shift in my ambulance. There is a huge difference between being a preceptor and a mentor. I remembered the hardships I saw other students endure with other crews and it wasn't the best learning environment. I would rapidly learn the students' personal challenges and they would learn mine too. I was a big teddy bear. Nothing was a secret when it came to personal strengths and weaknesses. If we felt like saying something, it was always said with respect and nobody ever took offence. It worked both ways as sometimes she would make me a little embarrassed when I crossed the line even just a little. But all in all, it was the perfect team.

Our unique bond was made over the time we made Sarah a better EMT student than any of our past students. We pushed each other to make her the best student in the world. We could see her passion. She shared our desire to help others; to stop their pain and make their day as well as it could be, just as I did. That was not only rare, but it was very unique. I'm sure Lisa approved, looking down from the heavens. The first tour was painful but we were partnered with another paramedic for the shifts, mostly for moral support.

The first few calls were very emotional but after the normal patient care got started, it flowed much better. Slowly the mentor medic stepped back and by the end of my last night he was not even there but bugging Sarah, while I did my job with passion. At the end of our tour I got a huge hug from both of them as I left the station. I looked up as I was walking out and the sun was shining. It was the perfect day to go for a drive to see the mountains after a few hours' sleep. As I walked in the door at home the happiest people on the planet met me even if they had four legs instead of the traditional two. I could not find a more loyal set of friends to greet me and care for me at home. I also knew my supervisors were making sure I was okay. Several times I saw them hanging around making sure Sarah was fitting in but they were also making sure I was okay. If I needed anything they would have stepped in and helped in a single heartbeat. They would not let me down as I wouldn't let them down. They to would not ever forget the horror with our crash and the aftermath. Anyone of them would have given up their life for either of us.

On my week off I finally made it to the mountains and was finally I was away from all pagers, phones or portable radios. My music never stopped playing unless I was sitting outside and my music was now the sound of silence. The therapy from being outside in the fresh air, even if it was cold at night, it was priceless. I thought about my last week back at work and then I thought of some of the calls we had with Sarah. I wondered why Lisa was spared from the hell on earth some days and I was still here, even despite the fact I should have died in the crash. Many times, I thought back and wondered if my life was an actual death wish off and on over the years. I had to have a purpose on earth, even if I didn't see it. I never thought of my role, as a paramedic as being heroic or extra special because all I was doing was helping people and that to me wasn't as special as people thought most days.

I sat and stared at the busy little river and watched the crystal-clear water running around the rocks and making its way downriver. If I tried to dam it up with rocks, it found ways around the rocks. Then I thought about my life and wondered if I was going up the river or down the river of life. The legendary salmon always made one last trip up the river. I thought about it for awhile then realized that I was more like a bear than anything. Then I wondered about some of the good and bad times of my life. I thought about the salmon again and wondered if that was my destiny. Did I want to die or did I want to live with the pain? That was my final question.

I haven't told anyone but a few times in my life I wanted to die. I just never wanted to complete the act or had a plan. I just didn't want to live in this crazy world another day longer. The fact that the pain was so intense, sometimes it seemed it was my only way out. I had seen many sides of hell on too many occasions. But I always got back even if I was just a little more scared or emotionally wrecked, even if no one really knew about my pain. In the end, I realized the pain gave me purpose. With purpose, I got recharged and refocused on my shaky road enough to keep going. My week off showed me that life had a purpose even if I was not sure what it was anymore. I went on down the road I was heading down.

Thank God, I got through the bad times in my life. Whether it was my guardian angel, one very good partner, possibly someone from the spirit world or just divine intervention, I was saved. Even if I wanted to die, I didn't get the opportunity and that was beyond my comprehension. Why? I may never know but the fact I was still standing today was reason enough for me. Just on calls I had been in serious trouble on five separate occasions and three times I could not get a second closer to having my birth certificate made into a useless paper. There must be a reason, so I had to accept it and keep walking ahead despite the intense pain some days, despite the tears and the heartaches. I had to go on. I just didn't know or understand why my partner was gone and why I was still in this world full of misery. Well they say misery loves company, so "here I am, my friend," I would say to nobody in particular. Bring it on.

On one of my days off I ran into my retired friend John the Pastor. John was a pastor for most of his adult life who and was one of the wisest people on the planet. John started being a pastor in the sixties in Chicago and had actually met Martin Luther King Jr. He survived the race riots and even worked as a pastor in the mental asylums which was pure hell, I'm sure. So, over the years he's seen strange stuff. But in his earlier years he also spent time in the war and has some truly amazing stories to share with me from time to time. We have spent many days together helping each other. When he needs help I'm magically available. When he needed heavy lifting, I was but one call away. My little Evan was like a winch truck because he was 6'4" and 320 pounds and when he lifted his share, my side got lighter as well. When John had a project that needed muscle, or he needed to move something heavy, we always found time to help him out. I could not have asked for a better friend. I had never met a kinder soul with a special link to my heart. My kids also got to see his wisdom, his good heart and his impeccable character.

This day I opened my heart to John. We had a standing rule that anything was safe to talk about. Work, play or personal life, it was all okay. We were having a coffee today on his deck off of his house and enjoying the heat from the sun, quietly watching the clouds pass. There are some quiet periods of just enjoying each other's companionship while our hot coffee cools enough to drink. John has an amazing aura around him. He can suck the evil right out of me after my bad shifts. After talking and sharing, it just seems to leave me and it's gone for good. After our visits, I seem to be able to sleep better, even if it's only for a short time. But sleep is sleep, generally overrated anyway.

Today I was all mixed up with emotions. I was depressed about life. I was glad I was alive but I was not sure why I'm still alive while multiple others I have worked with, including Lisa, are long gone. I have lost three co-workers over the last few years to suicide. Then I had two co-workers in the province that died young from complications of alcohol or drug abuse. I asked him why I was spared and why was Lisa taken. Why am I still alive? She was an angel in life and I was an old, hard, grumpy person, despite putting on a good show for others. Why do I keep going all while many others quit?

Looking back, I'd seen hundreds of others come into the EMS profession and they only lasted a few years. If the EMS field was their chosen profession, why did they leave it all? I go to work and do my best despite the problems. Why are they different from me? John smiled, held onto my shoulder firmly and looked into my eyes directly that were connected to my big heart. He spoke from his heart. John said:

"You were chosen for this work right from the time you were born. Maybe it was genetic pre-programming but I think you were in this right from the start. Many people in the EMS profession, the ones in healthcare and the clergy knew right from the start from inside your big heart this was right for you. Simply put, you have been chosen to help people for all the right reasons." By helping them you are fulfilling your destiny ironically as you are altering theirs but in the right way. Along the way the pain you are suffering from helping them is absorbed into your heart and you to must share their pain. The pain is something that someone must always bear but it's what you do with the pain that makes you a better person. If you take that pain and use it to push yourself to help others even more the pain is super therapeutic in a strange mythical way.

"I know I don't see you very often at church, but just the same, you live a Christian life. You can either decide to help the good side of life or support the evil side. It's your choice and always has been. We can fight evil and sickness with our hands and with our heart. You have a gift and your calling or gift is caring for others. Despite your mortal problems, you will feel the pain from others, but pain is not always a bad thing as it tells us we are alive. It tells us we still care enough to notice life and living. Just know you must keep going even when you have nothing left. I guess the analogy I like is when you're going through hell to help people keep going. Don't look left and don't look right.

In life always look ahead and no matter what hits you, keep going. If you're knocked down, get up. If you must crawl, then just crawl. In the end when you can't make it, Jesus will carry you back out of the hell you're stuck in. Many forget that part I'm sad to say. I wonder if that was why Lisa was your partner and together you never turned down the chance to help any people that were in need. You helped each other through the good and bad times. She was your guardian angel then and most likely today and forever."

"I have never shared this with you but many times after your bad days and after you went home, Lisa called me. Together we prayed for you and even though she never said it to you I'm sure she believed in you. More than anyone else on earth she trusted and loved you. She told me you were her guardian angel many times. I wondered as you now know, she was most likely your guardian angel all along too. Now from heaven she will always be at your side and will help protect you, I'm sure."

"Lisa told me about the time you had the very bad accident with the kids all killed and the parents also killed. Lisa called me and we shared the event. It was her time to let go of her pain. Lisa said it hurt you more than any other call you had ever done. The fact you had to throw the dead kids onto the dead parents was not something you can just forget as you retreated. Then you were forced to back off to a safe place while the firefighters fought the huge fireball. Knowing you had missed finding one little girl hurt you more than words can say. That missing child was so painful. Then the fact she was burned to death hurt your heart for a very long time. She told me it was so hard on you that for months you had nightmares. Lisa said you never told anyone about that one bad call. Even when she asked you about the call you just changed the subject and never talked to her about it again. You were not ready or willing to share the pain."

"She told me that you never said a thing about it bothering you. You made sure everyone on the crew was okay for days, but when you were sleeping you had nightmares. After that call, Lisa said you started working harder and even when any resuscitation was futile you would not stop. You would wake up sweating as if you were scared and the look in your eyes was pure hell for a second, then it was gone. We prayed for you together for we knew you could not or would not seek help, as that was not you." I looked at John and I could still see the fire, the bodies, the blood it was just like it was yesterday.

"Then one day you simply let it go and you were okay until the next bad one. She told me the next bad one was the pretty young girl hanging in her graduation dress. She said that one was so hard on you. You would never talk about it. Sometimes we can't or won't deal with pain until we are ready. Today you are ready and no matter what my plans are today, I'm not going anywhere until we are done." I looked at John and I said thank you with tears as that was all I could say right then.

So, for the next four hours we talked and the world never bothered us once. That day at Johns I cried, I wept for the lost, I wept for the ones we could not get to, and then I held onto my friend's heart and was nourished by his ability to give love without limits. Finally, I let my heart bleed until it could not bleed pain or hurt anymore. I had passed my hurt and my pain to my friend and with his superior inner power and strength he would bear my load at no cost other than being my friend. I would never know how someone could hold all that pain and be able to sleep at night. I'm sure John had his share of guardian angels and they would be the ones that would not back down from any source of evil. God, I could not understand how such evil and unrest lived in a world when we had people like John trying to help the world be better but evil was slowly winning the battle.

"Despite the pain, or the cost we all have a specific purpose and maybe you were more than gifted to help others," John told me. "You could not face the world by yourself. You needed a guardian angel at your side, my friend. I think you are still alive for a reason and Lisa will most likely be watching over you 24/7. I can tell by your heart you never thought you were even close to being an angel and sometimes you most likely think you are a bit rough around the edges, but life does that to good people sometimes. Inside you are still golden even if your heart is scarred for life."

John continued, "Some people have a special gift and despite the hardships it creates inside your heart, it's for a better reason than we will ever comprehend. You think about it and on the way home and I know you will understand it a little better. Even if you don't know why, you are alive for a reason, so know that it's a gift that you can't waste. You will get over this low point in your life and you will excel again. It will just happen when it's your time. You need to go home and sleep my friend. My home is always here for you with coffee anytime." I got a good long hug and thanked John for all his wisdom and kind thoughts. On the drive home, I thought about what he said and it started making sense to me. At one point, I stopped and I watched a small deer out in the field running around all while its mother just watched from a short distance. Somehow, we all needed someone to reach out over us and in my world, I was the fawn and John was the parent. My healing would come from the fact I knew I had someone to always be a friend to turn to when the world got me down. The day heaven took John I lost my one person who was always on my side and I'm sure over the years I got many a prayer with my name it from his kind soul.

After I got home I thought more about what he had said. Some days like today fate happens for a reason. "You're alive for a special reason," John stated. You have been chosen to help people. The way I see it, it's right from a message in the bible that makes me know one important thing. He said, "God would never give you anything you were not able to handle." We take the worst of the worst and make it better. We walk into any disaster and we come up with a plan. We try to save lives. We literally can stop suffering in seconds. That is a gift in itself. My gift of helping to heal or help others was also a gift from heaven. I was so fortunate to help anyone I could and for that I should be grateful.

As I sat back and realized I was thinking it was amazing that I could simply make miracles happen with our education and with my extra experience. If I can take a dead child and give them life if they are meant to live that to me is a miracle in the making. We can hold the hand of a dying lady and give her hope for her family. Lisa was meant to go to heaven. In some unique way, God or heaven needed her more than we did. My job on earth is not done. I needed to take the pain from losing her and turn it into a light that never goes out. I have the gift and the ability to share the gift with others and think about it like this: "I even get paid to help people." That's a win-win if ever I heard of one. After a while I thought more about my visit with John and started to smile to myself as just now I could realize "he's the real angel" and "I'm just his helper most days." I'm just the worker or helper of other people but that is just fine with me.

I'm okay with doing what I do but I also know the pain is eating me up. I need to deal with it as it comes up and make sure it doesn't destroy me too. Someway I will fight the good fight and save as many as we can. With the right partner, we will make a difference. At work and off work, I will help people. For every person that treats me wrong I will just walk away, and know they are not really bad, just they are full of pain and their suffering is much worse than mine. Someday they will be touched or helped but not by me.

On my last day, off before I was meant to go back to work I read a few short articles about different ways to deal with stress, pain and suffering. Yoga, swimming, walking and one new thing I came across which is unusual. It's called Mindful Meditation that comes from Buddhism where we focus on our breathing to remain present and in the moment. I decided I would need to research that to understand it better. But at least I could see the benefits of using it to help regulate emotion, increase learning and improve memory. Heck, I would do anything to help my grey matter improve. I needed all the help I could get most days.

Simply, you need to sit in a comfortable chair or cross-legged on the floor. You close your eyes and breathe; intently focusing on each breath you take. If your mind wanders or starts to wander, you bring it back. You can do it for up to five minutes and slowly increase it until you get to fifteen minutes, then you have mastered a good tool to help you relax. The hardest part was to get away from the stimulation of the world around you that makes it easy to be distracted.

The next way to relax made me laugh because I had no idea it even existed. It is the world of adult colouring books. My first thought was stupid as I thought it would be colouring nude people or something (it's "adult") but it gets better. You are actually trying to learn to colour and all you need to do is to keep inside the lines. You get better at keeping the colour inside the lines as you practise. It gets more intricate with increasingly complex pictures and patterns as you develop your ability. I wondered how I had missed this as it's been out for several years, though I had yet to see it or know anyone who practices it. That's when I realized I had probably worked too hard and too much and missed the relaxing parts of life. Now I needed more days to relax. I needed a long time to unwind after my shifts.

When I got ready for bed, I slowly realized the pains had been growing less and less over the last few days. My last six to seven months had been pure hell but every month things were a little better so it's not all bad. I would only take painkillers a few times a week and so far, sleeping pills were not needed so I can't really complain. Every once in awhile, I would have a few drinks with the right people in a private setting. However, I would seldom drink anywhere around my hometown in any public place. If I was having supper in plain clothes, I would only have one drink and I always had my back to the wall in every place that served alcoholic beverages. It was just a good habit to stay alive or out of trouble. I had seen many bad things and so often it always occurred in or around the use of alcohol or drug use.

I never thought it right for any professional to drink in public or wanted anyone who was a patient or co-worker to know or think I was human. It never looks good when you are considered the professional and you are seen buying and drinking alcohol where you work. I just knew too many people and I didn't want to let them down, so I was always on my best behaviour in all public places. The local police would never ever see me acting unprofessionally. I wanted to set the bar high for our profession. Even if I got pulled over and got a ticket if I deserved it then it was my fault. Somehow, I never had any trouble with the RCMP or sheriffs but radar traps or city police were mandated to pass out tickets and that was part of their job. Too bad they never figured out talking to people and working with them was a more effective communication tool.

I remembered an old work partner who I was called to, to try and get him off his quad. He was completely drunk and driving his quad in town. He was so drunk I could not stop him. I tried to reason with him. He was a volunteer firefighter and an EMT in the past. He told me off and I drove away. I lost a lot of respect for him that day. Afterwards, he got two impaired driving charges and lost his job, lost his family and slowly drank himself to death. He died at the age of forty-eight from the complications of his ETOH abuse. Looking back, I know for a fact it was PTSD and we never got him help. We didn't know what PTSD was back then. Sadly, he died a lonely death and when I went to his unannounced funeral there were not enough people there to call them mourners. I was asked to be a pallbearer at the last minute and gladly helped. I had forgiven him a long time ago for telling me to get the "****" off his driveway.

I just knew life had its up and downs for all of us. I was looking forward to visiting my friends on the east coast and sitting back and drinking a few beers, all while watching the ocean right in front of me. As I'm relaxing I can see myself buying a house off the ocean or building a house somewhere facing the ocean. In my mind, I was trying to figure a way to make it energy efficient as I settled into a long restful sleep. Tonight, the demons and the evil were not welcome. In my dream, I realized Lisa and John, my true guardian angels, were fighting them off so I could get some much-needed sleep. Tonight, it was just good dreams. Nothing bad was going to get inside my life as the blue sky keeps the darkness away and the bright moon burns away the evil from the darkness of the night.

Tinsel always had my heart protected.

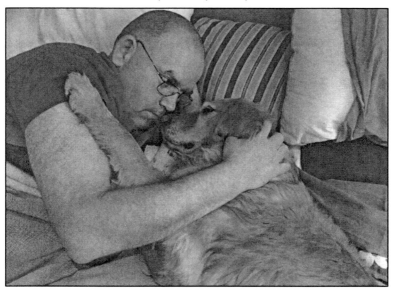

"On Our Worst Day, We Needed Each Other"

Chapter 6: Dying to Live

"Letting Them Come Back"

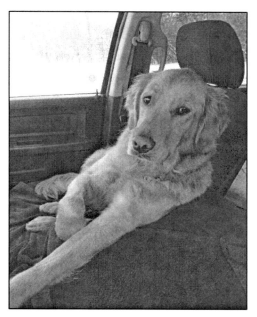

"Some Heroes Come with Four Legs"

Our day had been full of normal calls so far. We have just responded to our third sick person call of the day. It was the season of sick people and the winter was just getting started. We didn't mind the sick person calls as it was a call and it made the day go faster. Sarah was driving as I attended our 76-year-old female who had abdominal pain off and on for a week. I had just finished patching to the local

ER and they are expecting us in ten minutes. Just before arrival I give her an extra dose of Morphine 2.5 mg slowly pushed into the IV as she still has pain even after our initial analgesic medication was administration. I was careful not to give her too much but I wanted her pain manageable. I also wanted to make sure she was not going to vomit on the nurses so I gave her Gravol® 25 mg very slowly IV but diluted in 20 mLs of normal saline. I ensured the IV is running wide open to dilute it even more over a few minutes and then slowed the IV back down to keep the vein open (TKVO) in order not to cause congestive heart failure (CHF). It was what we called a very easy ambulance call but a real call just the same.

I knew she needed a little more IV fluid but it's best done over time in a controlled environment. For geriatric patients, it's often hard to guess what the real problem is in many cases. They often have multiple concerns and not everything makes sense so we try to get as much information as possible and pass it on to the local ER staff so they have as much information as possible. Many times, the hospital ends up doing a Chest X-ray and a BNP and finds our patients are in acute heart failure as well as have some element of dehydration. That was why it was best to initiate the most appropriate care and let the hospital continue or augment it on a case by case situation. I never once felt bad telling the local ER nurse I was not sure what was wrong but the patient was sick. Call it gut instinct and most often I was right.

My brain was sore today and I was not at my best today at all. I wanted to be at work but the day was not great with so many thoughts of the events from the last year flying around in my head. I must have not slept much at all last night. I was working through the stages of grief but couldn't get past the bargaining part and the depression part comes and goes some days. I missed the denial stage totally and don't know why. The anger part is a waste of time as there is no one to blame. God is off the hook. The devil was more likely but anger doesn't seem to fit. Somewhere out there I was trying to blame the system. People working sixteen-hour shifts, driving tired, texting and driving was likely what killed Lisa. But I know drunk driving keeps killing and no one follows the logic to stop it at all costs, so somewhere the system takes the credit. The acceptance part is not in reach, yet. I thought back to one fine RCMP officer killed on the Queen Elisabeth highway and the driver got off easy for he was tired. I'm sure his family cannot come to terms that that was an acceptable reason especially when he had already done the same thing in the past. Knowing that and knowing our corrupt justice system it all made sense. Sadly, it was the way the system worked in the modern world. The only saving grace was one other RCMP moved at just the right time that day and his life was spared but not the memory of watching his friend and co-worker die in mere inches in front of him.

I would have to work on my problems with my close friends. Getting some closure would help but I was not quite ready for that just yet. My brain needed more time to absorb it all, sort out my thoughts and arrange them in the right logical order. Having a bruised brain doesn't help my cause very much. The fact that I had repeated head injuries over the years plus the bad accident really made my brain angry with being shaken around way too hard. It made it harder to concentrate and to make complex decisions quickly. I used to be able to do multiple complex procedures half asleep, but not now.

I did some good research about the average complications and recovery from traumatic head injuries. Mine was most likely going to change me for life. If I added the four concussions over my life, it's lucky I can remember my name on some days. From my readings at BrainLine.org I remembered the part such as the headaches that do not go away being the most common complication in many post-injury patients. The difficulty remembering, or concentrating on simple tasks, or making quick decisions that we need to make, as a paramedic was not as easy. It was hard on anyone, even the people without a significant head injury. I was lucky to be alive and luckier to still be a paramedic.

When I figured out my feelings, it was like my brain speed was driving in a slow fog or in the clouds. I could not see what was in front of us and I didn't know when to turn or if I should just stop. Then I just hoped we didn't get hit from behind. I was slightly slower in my ability to think at warp speed. My ability to read was not as good today, but it had never been amazing. I found getting lost was easier. It seemed like north and south were mixed up or someone moved them around. I also noticed I became tired more easily some days but then I was half worn out to start with, so maybe it was normal. It was days like today that I wondered if I should have come back to EMS after the accident but it's my life. I had nothing else.

I had nothing else as a career that I wanted to do or could do so my options were limited. If I hadn't had such a great employer and an even better partner to watch my back I would have had to quit. I would have lost everything. If I could not work I would have no good reason to live other than my loyal golden retrievers, Pebbles and Tinsel. Everyone needs a purpose in life, or they are a lost soul. I know many military veterans actually live on the street and many have PTSD but society looks the other way. I was not going to end up on any street, begging for food or money to drink. That would not happen. I could not let it happen to me. Somehow, I had to walk down a different road even if the use of drugs or alcohol helped take the edge off the pain it never helped in the end.

Thank God, I had Sarah as a partner who made me feel at ease with the world. Nothing would have been harder than working with someone who failed the basic human communications course. Some days Sarah would finish my sentences when I was a little slower than normal and it made me happy to be with a partner that cared so much for me. She has become my guardian angel just as in the past we were once hers when she started in the EMS profession.

It seemed so strange how we ended up taking her on as a student with nothing but the desire to be the best and build her up to the present-day professional. Between Lisa and myself mentoring her, she became one of the best EMT's that I had ever seen. Then one day she was pulling me along out of the darkness and I was at a loss for words. It was so strange how life could take you from an all-time high and take your knees out from under you and you needed to learn how to walk all over again.

One time Sarah really saved my career, as I was going to drop someone or knock him into the middle of next week for being so evil and foul to us all. We went to a rollover with a drunk driver who was not nice to anyone. He was making me very angry for his rude comments to us all. He was rude to the police and they had to smile and nod all while we assessed him. Normally I can take it, but today it wasn't in the cards. Just as I was getting ready to knock him hard into the middle of next week, Sarah walked right in front of me and stood her ground. She just stood right in-between Mr. Obnoxious and me and took over my call. I actually wanted to go around her but suddenly I knew why she was standing in front of me. That was our unwritten rule between us both and I had done the same with Lisa a few times when Sarah was our student so that would be where she had learned that important step from in our past. It's called our personal intervention technique. So, I had to honour it.

Then he made the stupid mistake of suddenly punching her hard in the middle of her chest and my RCMP friends on scene took him out hard and fast. He made some very unwise moves at least twice that day. "You just never hit a lady" especially in the presence of a group of superhuman men. It's never a good idea to even to think about hitting a lady especially one trying to help you. I didn't even have a chance to intervene as I had caught her coming backwards toward me but thankfully I had caught her before she hit the ground. In seconds, he was face down on the ground and in handcuffs. His day to hurt someone else was over. Sarah was okay and thankfully uninjured. The RCMP even apologized but it was not their fault. Some people will never respect a lady or, respect a police officer, or follow the laws of our society. This was one day he should have tried to be nice and he would have sobered up in the ER and not in a local jail cell. Even better yet he should have never been allowed to drink and drive.

All in all, it could have been much worse. Heaven forbid he had hurt her or he would have had his birth certificate challenged. It's possible that he would have died of natural causes right then and there, I was almost sure for I'm sure I too would also make him regret his errors in a split second. We never had to deal with him after that second. Our call was immediately over. If Sarah had a chance she would have been able to defend herself but she had gotten too close in order to keep me out of trouble. That made me feel very bad. I told her I was sorry and she said it was still funny even if she got hit – it would not have left any marks. I gave her a high five and we went to the unit to finish the ePCR, then we were off the scene and seeking some more real action. Next time we both would stand a little further away from an unknown patient until he proved he could be nice.

We would need to buy the police member's coffee next time we saw them in the drive-through or take them a ten from Timmy's for helping keep Sarah safe. They had bought us coffee many times before, for helping keep them safe. We made many small gestures to each other especially after we knew each other had a bad day or after any bad calls. It was the least we could do for each other. After all, if we were to be a family and EMS was to be closer together with our police and fire services, we needed to always treat them with respect and with grace. We needed them to get through our bad days with us and they were always on our side even if it was never stated.

Our next call was paged out as a cardiac arrest at a local store in a nearby community. It took us fourteen minutes to get on scene. On arrival, the local volunteer firefighters were performing CPR on scene as they were the closest medical aid to be dispatched and they had an Automatic External Defibrillator (AED), which was lifesaving. We got a quick report of a fifty-year-old male who collapsed at the checkout, making it a witnessed cardiac arrest. They had already shocked him two times. They had five members on scene so the CPR chest compressions were going to be easier. Every two minutes they would automatically switch out. One of the members on scene was our supervisor and another an off-duty paramedic but today was a volunteer firefighter and another two were EMRs.

We had enough backup already on scene so we cancelled our second unit as they were still clearing up from a busy emergency call. They needed a break anyway and we could give it to them now as we had all the backup we needed in the world. Today we would even ask Greg to drive and then we could work the code knowing our lives were completely safe. Man could he drive – he was actually better than me as a driver and that took some real practice.

Today everyone will get a turn to do chest compressions for at least a few minutes before trading off which makes them all feel a little more needed. This is going to be interesting, as many times there is nothing to shock but today it looked more promising. After our next pulse check we see the Sp02 and ETC02 starting to register, so it's hopeful. Maybe today will be a better day. If we get a pulse back it would rock. Today we had the right team, we had just the right equipment, all we needed was a small miracle and it came from within someone broken or in dire trouble.

Sarah and one of the EMTs will insert an IV right away and I will follow it up with an Adrenalin® 1 mg preload IV push. The IV is already running wide open so it will be to the heart in seconds. We had a quick look at the monitor and could see what looks to be a ventricular tachycardia and which is better than ventricular fibrillation. I noted there was no pulse so it's therefore pulseless ventricular tachycardia by definition. The best thing was that our end tidal ETC02 was now registering at 22 mmHg with chest compressions so our team is doing the right things. The chest compressions were very effective. We just need a little miracle and then we are off to the races. The Angel of Death, you would lose this round if we had any say in the matter.

We grabbed the Amiodarone and I injected 300 mg IV push as well. We were going to hit him with 360 joules on the next shock. I wanted to see if the drug shock therapy was going to work so it was my way of testing the ACLS standards of care. We all know that biphasic was said to be better and this was the time to prove it. At the end of the CPR cycle we checked and we still have ventricular tachycardia with no pulse. I got the fire members to keep doing chest compressions as I charged the LP-15 and we got everyone to clear the patient. Once we have a ready signal from the monitor I nodded to the firefighter member and as his hands came off his chest I hit the patient with the most powerful shock we could administer. He immediately resumed his powerful chest compressions so not a second was lost. In no time, we had a positive ETC02 up to 36 mmHg and after about a minute I asked him to pause and just as I planned in my mind, a pulse was present. We won round one. Now the real battle started. We needed to get him stabilized and off-scene to the most appropriate hospital with a cardiac catheter lab that wants a patient. This patient was even more special as he had arrested so he was in more need for the cardiac catheter team than most patients at least in theory.

Time is muscle, and today our patient's heart needed a little help from others on a much higher pay grade than any of ours. A flight team would be golden and a quick visit to the ER in a city hospital would be appropriate until the catheter lab is ready. The cardiac interventional team with a good cardiac care unit (CCU) for a sleepover would be the next step in the chain of survival, today. The cold therapy that was helpful after a cardiac arrest could be initiated after he gets to the receiving hospital, as it's not easy to maintain in our environment–as there are too many variable factors. Our dispatcher calls back and STARS is already on a mission. We are going to need to transport to the closest Interventional Cath Lab Centre, which is forty-five to fifty minutes away. That is lights and siren transport and somehow the traffic would somehow know it was the right thing to make room for us as we went speeding past. Greg didn't know it yet but he had somehow magically volunteered to be our driver / pilot today. He would have to really watch out for the bad drivers and every once and awhile one would challenge us just to be rude.

We elected to load our patient immediately and do everything en route as it was wasting time staying on scene. We were blessed with a smiling volunteer who just happened to be a firefighter paramedic to drive, plus we would grab the extra firefighter EMR and we are off scene. The rapid response fire rescue truck followed us to retrieve the members as soon as we got to our final destination. I know their help is invaluable and in cases like this, it's a pure team effort. The local RCMP found the spouse and will bring her and a victim services member to the city hospital, which is an amazing act of kindness. Our patient is alive but not out of the woods just yet. As we flew light speed to the city I was writing the ePCR report and Sarah was monitoring everything and keeping me informed of any concerns. She was my eyes and my ears all while I tried to ensure I covered the documentation as good as it could be despite the bumps.

Sarah got an extra IV inserted and locked it off. It's for emergency use only, she said. I wish we had a Foley catheter with a temperature probe on it but we don't. So, I elected to wait until we got to the city hospital, then they could insert it to monitor output and core temperature. I carefully passed an oral gastric 14 French nasogastric tube after we were on the highway to drain the stomach contents but most importantly the extra air from the stomach from the pre-arrest ventilations. All in all, our transport goes very fast. Our team has done an amazing job and our transport was an uneventful and smooth trip. Thankfully our experienced driver was able to keep the speed a nice constant ride to keep us from being thrown around in the back like being at ball practice. We still were flying but it was like a jet without any stopping or turning motions.

I have worked a few days with other drivers that almost killed me from accelerating or braking so hard that my head hit the metal bars hard and I was almost knocked out a few times. Only once did I get mad and give my driver grief for driving like an idiot but he didn't care as he was a casual who hated his own life. It was his last day working with me and now he's a plumber, which is a completely appropriate profession for someone who lacks caring compassionate behaviour. Sometimes shit really does run downhill but at least it's his problem now and not mine.

As we walked into the local ER Sarah yelled, "Ventricular fibrillation (VF)" and the firefighter started chest compressions immediately as I immediately reached to push the right buttons to charge the LP-15. The combo pads are still on so it's going to be an easy fix; I hoped 360 joules was the right solution to this nasty lethal rhythm. As soon as the all clear was ready I nodded. Our firefighter came off the chest and the shock was applied in a mere second. I noticed it was still ventricular fibrillation as we started the CPR cycle of chest compressions again. We were directed to a resuscitation bed and a code was called for our pending arrival to the main trauma room. We elected to administer another 150 mg of Amiodarone while walking down the hallway to the resuscitation room as it had worked the last time with an immediate shock as well. As we rolled into the resuscitation room I charged the LP-15 and hit him with another 360 joules and suddenly he was "back" all-be-it with a weak pulse; regardless, he had a pulse again. We elected to do another minute of CPR just to keep his heart pumping a little better.

Call it the "human mechanical assist therapy." We have nothing to lose and everything to win in this case and today our actions were fruitful with one more life saved.

The ER doctor took over the care and I gave him a quick verbal report all while transporting the patient onto the ER stretcher. The C02 level was now up over 35 mmHg and his SP02 levels were around 94% so our perfusion level was more than adequate. I thanked our team of firefighters for the excellent extra help. I thanked Greg the pilot of our ambulance mercy flight and they were off back to cover their local communities. Then I gave Sarah a big high five and a long hug. We had saved a life twice today; it was meant to happen. Today life was changed for one person and one family was given hope. Despite his heart stopping a few times he is alive and to his friends, he is still in the running. The world was going to keep this good man for a little longer as long as the ER and then the cardiology staff could get him through the next forty-eight hours.

On the way home, we stopped and grabbed a Timmy's. I also grabbed a Pepsi® just to give me a little more of a sugar rush for my tired brain. Sarah volunteered to drive while I worked to finish the ePCR. Suddenly I stopped and set it aside. Today it would have to wait, because I was watching the road. I was not going to let my partner down. I could not live with myself if something happened to Sarah. I was more than happy to just sit back and relax. I would carefully watch the traffic meet us and then simply pass us without hitting us. Today I was the spotter for the sniper and I was watching out for the bad guys. I could spot them a long distance away. I would simply call them off and Sarah could deviate around them. Today nothing matters more than us getting home safe. I don't know why but today I was extra paranoid about making sure we were safe.

Sarah started to talk about the easy stuff first and it was just small talk. At first it was the weather, then it went to our emergency call and how it ran from my perspective. I told her it was amazing.

The teamwork displayed was some of the best I had ever seen. No one raised his or her voice, no one got excited, and everyone had fun while saving a life. Today's call was the ideal emergency call. We worked very hard all while doing everything we had practiced for years and perfected every step on many prior calls. Today was the test we all knew was coming and somehow, we passed with flying colours.

After we cleared the traffic and we were away from the city Sarah reached over and touched my hand and asked, "Are you okay?" I thought about it for about a minute and said to her, I don't know… I think sometimes I'm okay but sometimes I'm not. I knew that I could trust her and she trusted me so what we say stays in the unit. I wonder to myself over and over why Lisa had to die. I wonder, Why I was spared? Lisa had the gift of being a better person than I ever was. Lisa was so good at this job. She had such a close family. It just makes no sense to me at all. I'm at a loss about the whole world anymore. The evil, the stupidity, the way nobody cares about others is getting worse. The waste of life on the street with fentanyl use is on the rise and for what, I ask, it's just a quick high. I just don't get it at all. I also wonder how long I can keep doing this job? Sarah acknowledges my thoughts and says something I didn't expect. Sarah said, "The world gets what it deserves." I asked, "What do you mean?"

Sarah says "many people want instant gratification for almost every-thing, they want drive-through medicine. They want drive-through quick food and they don't want to be accountable for anything." Sarah went on, if people would stop and enjoy life, appreciate the sky, see and smell the flowers, maybe just maybe appreciate the people around them, then maybe life would matter more today than it did yesterday. If you listen to the news it's full of bad and the papers and the radio news are the same." I thought about what she said and she was right. I had never thought about it that way but we are in a throw away world. People needed to change to having pride, trying to deal with life and maybe if they worked harder they could appreciate the staff they had even more. Sarah was wise beyond her years.

In my mind, many people don't want to do the little things in life for others to make the world a better place unless they are rewarded. I asked, "What would make this world better?" She just looked at me and said so clearly, "Let's change it. Let's change the world. One person at a time. We can't change very much fast, but if we try and help people see a more positive outcome in life, things can and will get better. As a team, we can make a difference in people." I had to think a few minutes before I could respond. I looked over at Sarah and said, "Why not?" We have nothing to lose and the world to gain. We just had to come up with a way to change the world that would work.

As Sarah drove we both were thinking aloud. Now we just need a plan and we needed to start someplace that makes a difference. Between the two of us we came up with a little list and started to plan our idea to change the world. The points are simple but it's a start and today is better than yesterday if we are trying to help make it better. A few of the ideas come from the recent Readers Digest we had both read while waiting for calls, the rest would come from my random thoughts.

So, here's the "Ten Things" we came up with and I worked on them and wrote them down in a logical order. Everyone has merit. Everyone can stand alone.

1. *Appreciate the Little Things.*
2. *Make Significant Connections. Find good people and stick with them like glue.*
3. *Only Allow People that Matter into your Life. Bad people bring us all down.*
4. *Look Forward to Something Every Day. Look forward to something that is good.*
5. *Plan out Good for Tomorrow. Plan it today. Make it happen.*

6. *Deal with the problem at hand and then it's over.*
7. *Forgive and Forget. Life is much too short to hold grudges.*
8. *Never Let Someone Sucker Punch You Twice.*
9. *Giving Back to the World Can Help You Feel Better.*
10. *Pause your Life Daily and Count the Good Things You Have.*

Well we had to have somewhere to start. After I read it over a few times loud enough for Sarah to think about it we both agreed those ten are the right ones and even more, they are amazing. We just have to share them with others and find a way to make them all work in our daily lives. Somehow, I know we can make our lives better and thus help others be better. I also know the world is so broken but then we always knew that. We would have to change it one day at a time.

We vowed to share our ten new things to others to help them have a better day. You put it on the fridge and every day you can look at it and think about it. It's a start in the right direction to achieve a positive attitude and it's better than ignoring life and looking away. Somehow our destiny and Sarah was meant to be together. I started to think about a recent re-run of NCIS. I had recited the quote from time to time to my friends.

On one of my favourite episodes from NCIS – "Tim" states it so well to the world. From the conclusion of the episode "The Endgame" – Tim McGee says it so well that I too must share it with everyone. Its pure logic has merit and is very powerful.

> *Anyone can achieve their fullest potential.*
> *Who we are might be predetermined.*
> *But the path we follow is always of our own choosing.*
> *We should never allow our fears or the expectations of others*
> *To set the frontiers of our destiny.*
> *Your destiny can't be changed but it can be challenged.*
> *Every man is born as many men and dies as a single one.*

The little speech makes so much sense to me today. We are placed on this planet for one specific reason. The purpose is simple: to help as many as we can for as long as we can. The only way to make a difference in others' lives is to give them hope and guidance. Even if the world is getting slowly worse and society is lowering its standards we can still do our best to turn it around. If we can stop and just help the people around us it's a start in the right direction. The people in need right in front of us are our first priority and we will help them first. If only we help one at a time, it's a start, and we need to start somewhere. Tim from NCIS is a very wise man even if he is just a mere TV character. Tim wins my vote as a good man just the same. That one TV show taught me many valuable lessons that I could use in my own life.

Our full potential is doing what you do and our personal challenges we face together make us a better person. We have the ability to take the fear you have and change it into good. Our ability to help others changes their destiny in some way. Even if it's at the very end of a person's life it's a start or it's measurable to someone. It's a dream for some to help others or to get help. It's a living for others such as us in EMS helping people every day. Most days we go to work to have fun and they pay us well to make it through the day alive so it's a win-win for me and for my partner.

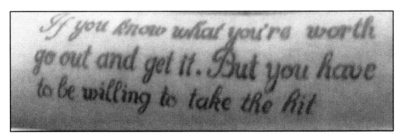

"Some days we just do our best and later on we deal with the rest."

Chapter 7: Taking One Too Many Chances

"Damned if You Do"

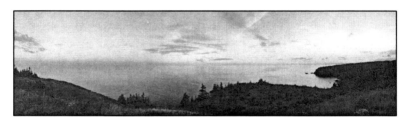

"Damned if You Do"

There is never a perfect patient; just as there is never a great set of protocols that works for everyone. We do our best with what we have. Sometimes good happens and sometimes bad happens despite our best intentions. One of the times that you think you're always right will be the day everything goes wrong just because it can. Today is one of those days. We are called for a sick person and the dispatch notes don't paint a very good picture for what we see on our arrival. As we were walking into the open door at the front of the house we saw the badness from the doorway. Sarah has the monitor and I have the basic ALS assessment bag along with the portable oxygen kit just as we have done many times on similar calls. We know this patient will need more than that but we will first need to assess our patient and make a plan of attack. In about a minute to ninety seconds we will have a game plan. Then our skills and our team will be put to the test one more time.

I almost laughed out loud as I thought about the art of trying to make a plan all while trying to deal with a patient disaster. It was funny as some day's we made a plan and it never worked so we came up with another plan. It was a game of chess and the chess pieces were real people. So, in theory we will plan as good as strategy as possible, but most likely an ever-changing attack plan will be the best case scenario. As we walked up to our patient, I thought this is a case of a very bad CHF or possibly pneumonia or, worse yet, it could be both. I don't have X-ray vision and our lab tests are very limited. The treatment for our differential diagnosis, if wrong, can kill our patient so we need to get it right the first time. Today the outcome is looking very bad at least for our patient. We have a backup unit if needed and they will gladly come and help us if we needed them but we had to make a decision right now either way. It is better to use them and if we are wrong it won't hurt our patient. I will be able to sleep a bit better tonight knowing we called them instead of the patient going into cardiac arrest without backup.

The dispatch history told us that we had a sixty-one-year-old male experiencing chest pain. But on arrival we hear the audible crackles from the doorway, plus he's breathing fast and looks to be in big trouble. He is pale and diaphoretic as well. We call for a backup unit or ask for a medical fire response to help. The patient is beyond sick. Over the years, we went off on main principle on our arrival at any sick or unwell patient. We needed to decide, "Sick or Not Sick" in the first several seconds of our arrival. Any level-of-conscious (LOC) problems, altered airway, bad breathing, or signs of shock are all we needed to trigger our "Spidey Senses." We are seldom wrong and if we are wrong the patient gets better treatment and a quicker hospital bed. Regardless, it's not something that they will use against us. Over the years, we have saved thousands so if we are wrong in one out of two hundred patients; it's an acceptable cost.

Sarah applied the LP-15. We applied the oxygen at high flow right away. The oxygen saturations were only 80% on room air, but worse, the C02 was also low which tells us it's most likely poor perfusion but could be from the rapid breathing. We got a temperature of 35.7 degrees Celsius which is more likely sepsis and not pneumonia. But shock can also cause the temperature to drop in decompensated shock. If only we could do a lactate level, we could guess a little more. The first BP is 74/44 which is not good. If we had the ultimate test we would most likely want a BNP which is Brain Natriuretic Peptide blood test but we don't have the luxury of it today. Upon arrival at the local ER, the staff physician will most likely add it to the required laboratory test. But we need to get the patient there alive first and foremost, before getting worse.

The first 12-lead says ischemic heart but nothing else is certain at this time. I asked Sarah to cycle the BP assessment every five minutes. Our LP-15 can automatically repeat a 12-lead if it notices the ST segment changing, so it's a lifesaving feature in itself. So far, I'm not sure but I think it's most likely acute CHF so I decided to try oxygen at 12 lpm via a non-rebreather mask (NRB), start an IV TKVO which basically is slow enough to keep the intravenous fluid flowing fast enough so it won't clot off.

I add some Ventolin and Atrovent just in case there are some acute COPD issues' as it will only help in most cases. In no time, our backup is walking in the door with our stretcher. I noticed the Sp02 is about 85 to 88% which sucks with high flow oxygen. I decided to initiate a 250-mL bolus of normal saline which, if it's pneumonia, will help with the BP but with some cases of CHF can make it worse. I asked our second crew to set up a dopamine infusion drip right away.

We could get a Foley catheter inserted as soon as possible but it's not likely until we get in the unit, as it's not the biggest priority. Our patient is about 110 kg so we'd best titrate the right amount of medications as giving medications weight-based is better than a generic dosage. We need to try and be accurate in our weight estimate to initiate the dopamine infusion at the correct dosage as well. Most days it's an educated guess.

In the worst-case scenario, the local ER staff will do it if we run out of time. Our goal is to try and get the BP over 100 systolic so a nitro infusion can be started, but as of yet our patient's BP is still too low. If it's pneumonia, Lasix and nitro can cause the BP to crash so my head hurts thinking about all the options. In no time, our patient is in the unit and we are off to the local ER. Our patient is looking better, but not by much. The BP is only 88 systolic so I initiate the dopamine infusion at 5-mcg/kg/min, which today is 550 mcg/minute, and we will titrate as soon as we get an accurate BP after the medication has had a few minutes to kick in.

I was praying the heart wasn't very irritable today, or the dopamine might make the heart rate irregular and even cause it to go into ventricular tachycardia or just beat too fast to be effective. So far, it's only slightly faster and the hospital is in sight so we elect to leave it at our initial setting. I was not aware someone patched the ER but not sure who did, as I was a little busy.

I just wished my head wasn't so foggy but today it is and it hurts just to keep focused on the current problems despite the need to think hard on the other potential concerns. I was so happy to see the BP of 102/66 and a Sp02 over 92% as we rolled into the trauma room. Despite the respiratory rate of 28 to 32 breaths per minute it's looking better than when we started. There is nothing worse than being acutely short of breath (SOB) other than being in severe pain, I think to myself.

The ER staff is ready and waiting for our arrival and I knew our patient was in good hands now. I knew as soon as we get past the automatic doors our patient's care is going to be better than what we can provide on most days. Not all days, but most days it is the best place to be if we are in trouble and having trouble staying alive. The emergency room staff have a few tricks up their sleeves we can only dream of.

As we give the report we notice the lab and X-ray staff are ready and standing in the corner, which makes me proud to know our doctors trust us so well with our initial differential and the doctors have the same concerns to rule out or rule in. Soon we will have a definitive diagnosis. As we stepped out of the room, the portable chest X-ray (CXR) is already being set up. In no time, the second IV is in and the essential labs are taken; in twenty to thirty minutes they will have a complete lab picture.

The physician immediately draws an arterial blood gas (ABG), which is a great idea as it can give them the electrolytes, a lactate and blood pH in a just a few minutes. The CXR shows the doctor bilateral infiltrates and fluid, so pneumonia and CHF are very likely. The BNP was also over 1000, which is positive for acute CHF and the troponin is slightly elevated. The slightly elevated troponin is most likely heart strain or a type 2 acute myocardial infarction is likely, so not a big deal but it completes the picture.

Today this patient is being admitted to ICU and his family are called to stay at his side as his next few days are going to be scary for everyone involved. I was just so happy today with the staff working with us. The ER staff and the other staff all worked so well – I know that teamwork made the outcome even better. This is one day that everything worked out but not all days go this well. I have seen days when no one seemed to work well with each other and the outcomes were terrible. The call was a good example of us not knowing what should be done for a patient.

Sometimes there is no really good way to know which pathway is the best and sometimes the only thing we should do is almost nothing. Once we start down the wrong road things can slowly get worse and despite our best intentions we make things worse.

I think back to the cases where I was almost convinced of the problem but someone or something told me to stop. It's almost like making a lethal drug error and for some strange reason you stop at just the last second. Just when you think you're amazing, or superman, the world can find a way of knocking you back to reality. I thought back to one time I was going to give potassium chloride in a 1000 mL IV bag and I was so tired I almost injected it into the patient instead of the bag. It would have been a very painful and terminal outcome even if it was an accident.

It's a wise decision to always remember that if we are not sure what to do we can always call a friend, which in our case is the online medical control (OLMC) or the local ER doctor. In many cases they have guided us to the right care or steered us away from creating a medical disaster. In many cases over the years I have had to ask friends or my local medical director for advice while doing a call and they are more than happy to help a friend in need. I know sometimes in the past we really made an effort to help and despite the attempt, the patient still decompensated.

Someway or somehow, we needed to help Sarah and our future students to be better practitioners and hopefully make fewer mistakes even if sometimes it's part of the care, we provided. Sometimes our actions can have iatrogenic effect which is from the Greek for "brought forth by the healer or professional" that really refers to any harmful effect on a person, from any activity of one or more persons acting as healthcare professionals trying to help or while providing medical care.

Just know that with all the knowledge and all the wisdom in the world you can't always be right in providing just the right care. The mistakes are educational, as long as it's not a negligence concern on our part. We need to think on this and somehow, we can make this world a safer place or create a better profession in EMS or in the emergency room. Over the next week, I will review some literature and surf the web for some electronic suggestions. It will make the decisions easier for our co-workers. Maybe there are better ways to make the diagnoses more accurate and with less chance of human error, I would hope. Just thinking back and I know that almost fifty percent of pharmacology errors are system errors.

After our call is done we are back at the base waiting for the shift to finish. I just happened to run into one of the other senior paramedics and she asked me for a little advice in life. I was not sure what it was about, but I said sure. I suggested our unit where we could sit and talk privately. On the way, we both got a coffee and took a seat in the front of the unit. This way we can watch the CAD and we will know before anyone of any pending calls. Old habits die hard. After all it's our personal office but on six wheels and it's about the only place we both feel safe to talk freely.

Bobbi has been one of my friends for years but I don't work on the same shift with her often unless one of us is covering for someone else. I know her as a very quiet but good medic. Over the years, she has seen hell here on earth. I respect her greatly, for we have fought many personal but intimate battles saving the dead or very close to it despite the odds. Today I have someone I consider an equal to talk to no matter the reason she needs to talk and it's someone that she trusts to be on the receiving end. She is considered one of the good senior medics and she is trusted by everyone at work and in the ER for any emergency care.

Bobbi thanked me for the time to visit. I asked her what was up. Bobbi looked at me and said, "I'm having trouble. I lost my mom last year and my dad is not well. I miss my mom and since she died, Dad is slowly quitting." Bobbi continued, "It's just like someone shut his light off. I call him lots, but it's not enough. He has no one and I have no other family so it's my call. Dad needs me now and not later. I think I should take time off but I don't know if I can come back if I leave. I'm so ready to retire and if I leave it's my way out but if I stay, I miss time with my dad." "Where does your dad live?" I asked.

Bobbi replied, "He lives back east on the coast and I'm too old or too tired to start over in a new province. I just don't want to start at the bottom again. My career is almost over as a street medic but I can't afford to retire just yet." I thought a bit and magically I had an idea. Maybe destiny has a solution, even if I never saw it coming for me. It might help others and today was a possible good outcome in the making.

I said, "Well maybe I can help you with this little problem. My friend works in management in Newfoundland and I was talking to her just last week. They have a few special job openings for a manager with a vision for a new "Community Medics Program." It's a unique job and she is looking for a few special staff to get it going." When my friend told me about it I declined as I'm not much into the palliative issues as I was not into seeing more people die. I have seen so many deaths over the years it is one part I can't or won't do willingly anymore. Heck, I don't even go to funerals anymore. Since losing my partner it's not something I ever want to think about again. I'm still not ready to say goodbye to Lisa even if it's what I still needed to do.

Somehow, for some strange reason I needed Lisa at my side right now. Someday I will need to deal with it but I was not ready to say goodbye just yet. Even if it's eating a hole in my soul, I can't really let it go, even if it's what needs to be done. Somehow, I knew I should or that I had to say it but I was not ready. Someday, I will need to cross that road sooner than later but it would need to wait a little bit longer. I just could not face saying goodbye, even if it was a long time ago.

I looked at Bobbi and knew there was a possible solution. Knowing Bobbi, it would be a great position, as she loves the special people in this world, that's not all blood and guts related. It's dealing with the less fortunate, the people with no fixed address, no real outlook in life but the next drink or the next fix. It's not my world but that's okay. I looked into Bobbi's eyes and I could see her heart shining through them. Then I thought maybe she could retire in her home province and it made me smile even more. I said, "Bobbi, it's an idea." Slowly I can see her starting to smile inside. She can see the future. Even if it's not what she expected or wanted, it's a way out.

I then had a special surprise for her. I reached into my pocket and phoned my friend. She's on my speed dial list as she is one of my PTSD emergency support contacts. This is not an emergency but it's important just the same and I know she will answer the phone everytime I call. In fifteen seconds, I have a smiling friend that's over 3,000 kilometers away at the other end. I just made her day even if she's worried about me just the same. I first told her I was okay and in a minute, I conveyed how I was really doing but had to change the subject and tell her of my special request. Then I passed the phone to Bobbi. In no time, they were talking about the good people of the world.

Something about the east coast people I still can't get over is how they are so good to others, no matter their past or their reasons for needing help. A good example is they don't or won't take payment for helping people in need. After a trip staying with a few of them, I came home and had a renewed hope for mankind. They have life figured out, despite being just a little poorer than the rest of people in my world. Many of them have seen hardships but not a word was ever said about it, nor would you ever hear them complain. They truly are the salt of the earth and they care deeply about others. They don't need to lock their doors and they use the honour system. Better people in the world would be hard to find.

They mean it when they promise to lend you a hand. If you needed help you just called and they're already coming over. It was a simple but effective way to intervene, a way most had forgotten about.

This was something I remember that was common among our farming community in Saskatchewan. When a neighbour called for a hand you dropped what you were doing and you went and helped them out. Just as they did the same to you when needed.

As I sat in our ambulance my thoughts went back to one of my darkest days. A flashback to many years ago, when we had lost too much all too fast. I had nowhere to go and no one to turn to that would not make me feel even worse. I was sitting in my room and I was ready to say good-bye to the living. I had seen so much tragedy and then personal fate hit me even harder. No matter what I tried to do I could not see light. Over and over I could hear the screams from the dying kids and the parents that were left alive, but it was beyond screaming. It was a call we had done several years back when another drunk driver had wiped out a big family and he somehow lived. I guess he lived with the guilt despite a soft jail term but the kids got life and it seemed wrong to know he got away with killing them and that their parents' lives were changed forever.

On our arrival, the fire was just starting to get going. The fire crews were right behind us but not quick enough as the propane-powered vehicle went up in a fireball in seconds. The fire was knocked down but the screams never stopped for days in my head. Multiple EMS and firefighters quit after that bad night, long before anyone realized they should have been helped out. Some of them were labelled "quitters or burnouts" for the wrong reasons.

We didn't know about PTSD, or formal or informal debriefing. We did not participate in the critical incident stress management (CISM) process. We had no idea compassion fatigue was so relevant to EMS and health care workers. We had no idea that no matter what we do after the fact, we are still affected for a long time to come. We can't easily just forget the tragic events and make it go away with a debriefing. Counselling and special one-on-one sessions are often the best way to deal with the severe cases of PTSD. Sadly, they were rare or not offered at all after the most serious calls. That was most likely why we had lost so many first responders as it was all the bad calls building and it just took one more bad call to make it too much to bear. It's often not one tragic episode but more often multiple events that occur all in a short period of time.

Thinking back no matter what we did, the sights, the sounds and the smells stayed with us forever. Then for some people things kept getting worse. Then it all came to a "no way out" that terrible night, all I could think about was to be making it stop. I had the gun and I had the bullet. All it would take was one. But I could not do it. I had called my friend and after an intervention and a long holiday I came back and went back to work but I was not the same for a long time. I was so close that night to pulling the trigger and taking my chances; but in the game of life, Russian Roulette had dealt me a losing hand. I somehow beat the odds. Just maybe my guardian angel had my back that night. More likely a few more were also at my side for backup.

I simply walked away with nothing left and made it out with nothing but my life. It was not until I was in a safe place with a friend that I finally broke down and the evil from many bad events came out. They came back all at once and slowly we broke them down to one bad call after another until they all came out. Still today sitting in my unit my hair stands up just thinking about how close I came to be walking down the wrong path of life. Thank god, I got a second chance to face life and received a second chance to live again.

This is one of the real reasons I go out of my way to help others in trouble in my EMS profession and with all people in general. Everyone should be entitled to have a bad day. In life, we might only get one chance to help people in need. No matter how trivial the problems others might be having, we can always stop what we are doing or pull over and help people out in times of need, if it is safe to do so. Every once in awhile, we might get a strange feeling that it might not be safe, then we must keep driving. We need to call it in, but ensure the people coming with backup are also safe. We can give them a vehicle description or licence plate if at all possible. It is helpful to describe the people that were on scene that might help make the approach plans safer for the police. We just don't want them walking into a trap or an unsafe situation.

We need to make sure the police get any extra chances to stay out of harm's way, if at all possible. From what our past has taught us some people want to do harm to others for no other reason other than they can. The past police killers in Mayerthorpe, St. Albert and Moncton proved that nowhere is it safe for police, firefighters or EMS when we are trying to help others in need. No matter where we live, evil is close by and lays in wait to cause harm to others that might least expect it. We need to increase our situational awareness to ensure we all are kept a little bit safer while at work. We need to make sure our co-workers go home safe at the end of the shift.

You would think helping people should be easy and straightforward, but it's not always that simple. Most times we are rewarded in kindness, but sometimes the true nature of evil people comes out. Some people are abusing the system, using people or abusing people, but this isn't our fault. The fact is that over time we will end up helping thousands in need and be burned or harmed by only a select few but unfortunately that is the acceptable price of helping others. After all, it only takes one person a mere second to change our destiny just as we will try to intervene in our patients medical or trauma events. I'm just thankful that most shifts we help more good people then the thankless ones.

By helping people in need, we make the world a better place. By helping Bobbi, I had made her years of helping others even that much more special. To simply pay it forward works in our favour in most cases, and it paid off triple today. Today destiny helped Bobbi and made me remember why life is so precious. It's been a good day no matter the sleep we lose thinking about the issues that just don't stay away. Sometimes we need to simply count our wins in life and let the losses be as they were but lost from the very beginning.

After about twenty minutes Bobbi hung up and passed the phone back. Today I helped someone that needed and appreciated the help. I had turned someone else's emotional or troubling day into a good day. Today I made someone know they counted. Out of the corner of my eye I could see the tears coming down her face. She isn't looking at me so much as she is looking ahead. Now she has a way out – the right to walk away. It will help her dad and in the end, it gives her a way out with grace. It's a win-win other than we will need a new paramedic sooner than many thought. That's okay as there are some keen young medics looking for more hours and soon they can be in her spot. On my next trip, out east I will have a new place to stop and visit a lifelong friend.

In a few minutes, she turns to me and she is beyond happy even if I'm the only one who sees the tears. She's still crying as she reached across the CAD and hugs me. Today my kindness helped a lady who has helped people all her life despite the cost to her soul. Today she has a way out and her dad will have someone at his side as soon as she hands in her notice and packs her bags. The good thing is my personal friend out east made a new friend today as well and today my friends are all that matters to me. Sometimes money isn't the reason we live and a pension is no good if no one is with us when we get to our final destination to relax and enjoy life. Today the hell on earth was turned upside down. Even if it's just for a little while, it's a start. Today the sunset is better than it has been for weeks. The glow from the sun is warming up the heavens. Today the good side is winning a little bit of lost ground. Today my friend is finding new light at the end of a long dark road.

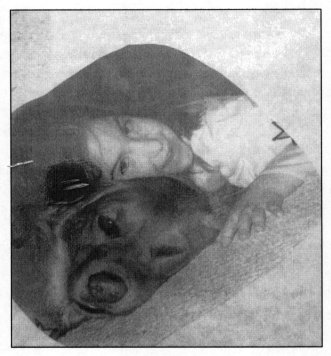

"Love Saves Lives"

"Life is too precious to waste and the more pain we see the more it matters"
"No Matter how many we lose the ones we save must help equal the debt"
"Even if it doesn't really add up it needs to count"
"After all, even one life is worth the cost"

**My inspirational message comes from the movie
"The Guardian" (2006)**

(The take-home message is to use our gift to help as many people as possible. We are all accountable to do our best once we become professionals. We can't change destiny some days, but we can affect the outcomes of the many events we come across).

Ben Randel said to Jake, *"You have a gift, Jake. You're the best swimmer to come through this program, hands down, by far, and you've got a whole record board to prove it. But you know what I see when I look at it? I see someone fast enough who's going to get there first. I see someone strong enough who's going to last. I see someone who can save a life maybe no one else could. You really want to honour them initials on your arm? Then honour your gift. Save the ones you can, Jake. The rest, you've got to let go."*

Save the ones you can, Jake. The rest, you've got to let go. That was the message I had to know in my heart.

> **"We too must do our best and let the rest go. After all it's all we can do."**

Dale M. Bayliss

"Saving them from Hell"

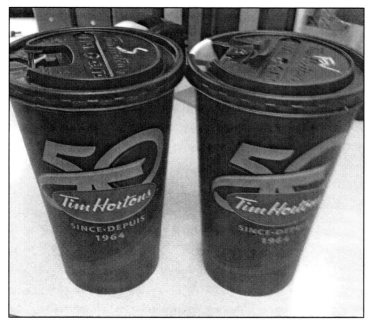

"Our Real Lifesavers Some days"

Every once in awhile, we make a difference by helping people. Last week we made a difference for multiple patients but some days we're not so fortunate. I would think that every once in awhile, we need to lose a tough battle or we need to put up a good fight trying to save a life to appreciate every actual life we save that much more. No matter how hard we try to win, we lose our share of medical or trauma battles. No matter how much we race to defeat the odds, the "Angel of Death" comes knocking and some days we must lose. What hurt the most are the battles when kids are lost, or the innocent are taken before they've had a chance to live. Some medical battles hurt more than others. Sometimes karma is the winner but not very often. I don't know why but good people seem to keep paying the price for the evil people around us all.

Today Sarah is driving us downtown for a much-needed coffee break. I'm trying to get my act together as the last few days I've lacked enough sleep. No matter what I do or try it won't work. I look over to her and can't help but admire the energy from within, the determination, the pure drive from inside not unlike me some twenty years ago. I just got my hot coffee and used my Timmy's card to reward my partner's superb attitude. I was so happy and thankful that today I had just the right partner. My first sip is very rewarding. But today the coffee is going to cool a bit more than we both would like. Today work is calling and time is not something we can alter or slow down.

We are paged out for a single vehicle rover. Coffee will need to wait. Today lives are counting on us and I'm counting on my partner's wisdom and skills to keep us both out of trouble and alive. We both would settle for the chance to let the less fortunate live even a little bit longer. Someone is having a bad day if they have rolled. Many of us like our job, but don't need to see any more accidents. When we are called, we will go and always do our best.

No matter the end results, we will fight fate and try to alter the destiny of the less fortunate. We will use our skills and our good pharmacology selection of our special medications; all the wisdom of every rescuer will be challenged. Today our team is going to be the right team. It has to be because it's all we have so we must make it work. No matter the outcomes of today, the chance to affect destiny or make significant changes in others' lives. It's on our shoulders, with our crew's ability to make life a little better for the people in need of BLS or ALS care. With our fantastic team approach every situation we face has a better outcome.

Today the battle for life is on and we will do our best no matter what the outcome is for our patients we will do what is right. Sarah is determined to get us to the scene safely so I can try to relax and think about a plan of attack on our arrival. Our second unit is coming in hot from the north. The accident is just off of the highway west of town and close to the overpass where the two highways meet. It's easy to find because it is east of the overpass. Jim and Tina are in Medic-Three and will be on scene just around our arrival as well. They are a great crew so we know our backup is the best of the best – so that is one less worry today. They are coming down the four-lane highway with extra police fighting for them for the chance to get to the scene first. Today the police will have their work cut out for them during the rescue but also after the patients are long gone for the investigation phase.

We are updated en route: there are three patients and we have additional units that are coming; the local fire is also sending lots of equipment and help. With the RCMP we should have all the help we need. The only other question is should we call for a helicopter early? If we needed or wanted STARS to auto-launch we could do it now and not be in any trouble. It was just we still don't have much information to go on. If we had a clear picture I would say yes, but launching them is never without risk. They have a very good record for safety but still, what if something went wrong elsewhere and we didn't even need them. Using them was an acceptable risk today. I would often launch them early but today something kept telling me to wait.

Then part way to the scene we are updated by dispatch of a possible fatality, which makes our urgency to get to scene even greater. We asked STARS to be on standby for now, as we now have a good reason to fly them just on the mechanism of injury (MOI) involved. Often, they would be pulled out of the hanger and already doing the preflight start up as we called for help. If one person is dead then the others are all most likely to have serious injuries as well.

Sarah subconsciously listens to my thoughts and she gives it a little harder than before. Our unit can't go any faster. I simply reach over and thank her knowing she has reached our maximum warp today. She looks at me and smiles back, knowing our thoughts are synced. "You're welcome," she says. I smiled back thinking this is a real team. It doesn't get much better than this. Too bad we don't have a student or a ride-along today. That was the only thing I thought we could use that we didn't have as an option. But after the query of possible fatality I immediately thought maybe John my retired pastor friend should be on this call but he's a long way past the prime of his life to be seeing this type of tragedy. We are all too old for that part most days.

As we approached the scene we found two vehicles crashed with one patient lying across the roadway. One patient looks to be still in each vehicle. Sarah tells me she will take the one in the closest car and I got the ejected one as a present. Most often the ones trapped in a vehicle where are less likely to be injured. Being ejected makes the chances of being hurt many times more likely. The other crew just radioed us that they would take the other patient in the second vehicle as they were separate crash sites. It looks like they crashed and then went flying until their forward was lost.

The first of the multiple RCMP vehicles are just pulling up and one member quickly puts their cruiser sideways to stop people from running over one of the victims. We have done the same on the other side of the unfortunate patient. That is excellent teamwork, I think to myself, and I know today is looking better already. We thought our other unit would beat us to scene but we won the race.

Today that was a bad idea. Thankfully our backup was just pulling off the highway.

I jumped out and grabbed the airway kit, Sarah takes the trauma kit. Basically, we both have enough to start to work on anything, but the second crew will help make it an even attack on the injured. Ben, the Corporal arrives on scene, walks over and tells me they have two more patient still alive, one in each of the vehicles in the ditch and one is very bad.

The one on the road is the deceased one and he's not our responsibility anymore other then we need to ensure he truly is dead. I took one quick look at him and pronounced him from about ten feet. After being ejected he most likely got his head crushed, which is good enough for me to consider being a lost cause for today. Dead is dead and we have two more living patients that will take all we have despite wanting to help everyone. Today our score is minus one and two people on first base. The rest is up to destiny and our combined team effort. "Shit" I said out loud as I just hate losing but today it was already in the cards of this person's life. Today losing is just part of the cost of people making the ultimate mistake and living for one person is not even an option.

The dispatcher calls back and tells me STARS-3 is in the air already and the estimated time of arrival (ETA) is about fourteen to eighteen minutes, which ultimately makes our day better. They have a doctor on board, which is a good backup for critical care air medicine as long as they are part of the team. I had a quick look at the second patient and realized he was a mess. Our second unit had just parked on scene. Backup does not get any better than that. Jim is a paramedic and Tina is a great EMT currently in paramedic school so they are better than most crews as they are very eager and dedicated staff. They walk over to me with their kits and monitor right away. I ask Tina to help me with the messed-up patient in the second vehicle and get Jim, the experienced medic, to go and help

Sarah. We are going to make Tina an honorary paramedic. Today she is an equal and we are her backup. We will work together on the other patient.

The firefighters are setting up a hose line just in case of an active fire, plus setting up the extrication tools needed, with an extra member helping with traffic issues. Fortunately, they have a few extra people to help us today. As we try to assess our patient with limited access, we notice a very injured patient with a severe facial smash and snoring irregular respirations. Today we can't do much patient care as the vehicle is smashed in around him. Today fire will cut him out and then we can try to save him.

I hope Sarah and Jim's patient is better off but both vehicles are mangled so it's not looking good for anyone today. I have a quick look and it looks as though the firefighters will have to remove the driver's door and part of the roof to access our patient. I decide to set up for an intubation in the unit. We have applied high flow oxygen and I know once the patient is supine, our airway is going to go straight to hell. So far, Tina has suctioned the blood out of the airway as best she can but it's not a good airway. Tina can't get to the patient and he has refused the OPA insertion so it's going to take medication to achieve a secure airway. Therefore, a chemically induced airway or a cricothyrotomy is going to be our alternative backup plan. Today we just declared war on trauma.

A backup BLS crew has also arrived and will help out as needed. They are an inter-hospital transfer service but today they are still backup. We get them to split up and we have Ben, an EMT helping us with Mike an EMR helping Medic-Three. Slowly the patient care is getting done. We have an emergency large-bore IV in for the RSI and we have a stable set of vital signs so any medications we want can be used today.

Fire is going to be another five to ten minutes despite working fast, before we can extricate the patient. Jim comes back and says the other patient is stable but needs to head to the city ASAP. He has internal bleeding but is awake, fortunately he has a good airway and has been stable so that's a good start. It's time to make a plan. I ask Jim if they are okay to just take Mike and suggest they just leave and bypass for the city. They will have a trauma team waiting for them and time is everything today.

I could see that Jim is a little worried about our patient but I told him the aircrew can help us and they will also take him to the alternate trauma hospital today so both patients will soon receive better care. We can also get Ben to bring the BLS unit and retrieve his partner as well if needed. It's a good plan and it works. Jim yells at me as he takes off to help Sarah. "Be careful, kids, save a life." Some days our teams need to split up and today is split as even as it can be to save two lives. Jim knows I've had some bad days and he is extra supportive towards me. He's got my back and I have his no matter the why.

I grabbed my mike and got an information patch to our dispatch to update the inbound flight crew. They are also getting a trauma centre ready for Medic-Three's patient. The air medical crew have been briefed that they will be needed to help with a bad airway on their arrival. They will be ready to go to war as soon as their skids hit the ground. They are already in the distance coming in low and very fast. Soon I can actually hear their rotors bringing them in safe and dropping into a quick orbit around our scene to look for hazards. God only knows how the sound of the jet engines gives me extra hope today.

The highway is quickly closed off and the fire crews are waiting to give STARS a secure scene close to us and just off the overpass. I get Tina to run to the unit and get the medications, the IVs set up and the monitor ready for the patient. Ben and I have a c-collar on already and a long spine board ready to help extricate the patient; as soon as he is free, he's ours. Our team is ready; even knowing the airway sucks, it's still our job no matter how difficult. We have our stretcher ready and the fire crew knows the plan to extricate to the unit as soon as humanly possible. I notice the breathing is becoming irregular and I know time is already against us. The STARS-3's crew is just hitting the ground when the patient is finally free. "Time to earn our bucks, my friends," I say, thinking out loud.

When fire has his body free we perform a rapid extrication and quickly we are wheeling the broken mess of a patient on our stretcher to the unit, the aircrew meets us and helps us put the patient into the unit. They have a very experienced flight paramedic, Howie, and a cool ICU nurse, Rachelle, who has been flying for years. Today they have an ICU staff physician who is also an anesthesiologist flying with them for some extra flight experience. Today the STARS doctor is going to get to show his stuff to the rest of us in no time but today his office is now in our unit. The equipment is not as fancy, but it works. Today our broken facial-smashed patient is almost lucky. Fate got the right team to come to his unfortunate circumstances.

As we loaded the patient, everyone is assigned roles and everyone has a job. Today my job is to get a second IV running and ensure the monitor is on and ready. The flight nurse is checking medications with Tina. Howie and the doc are getting ready to intubate with a bougie and the video laryngoscope. The airway is a mangled mess. They have a surgical cricothyrotomy kit sitting beside them if the worst airway today becomes unmanageable. The initial oxygen saturations are only 90%, which isn't good for high flow oxygen but it could have been zero. The C02 levels are high which means basically a terrible airway with poor ventilations, not a big surprise.

Howie is suctioning the airway again and attempting to ventilate a little better than before but it's going to remain a bad airway. The ventilating rate and tidal volume are so important to preserve life and to save brain cells but also very difficult in this patient due to the extensive facial trauma and already swelling of the normal facial features. The physician is checking the advanced airway equipment and getting ready for the first intubation attempt. The correct medications are being pushed in the IV tubing right now as the intravenous lines are running wide open. The time to get the airway secured is just around corner. The experienced physician says calmly and clearly, "Let's get it done."

Everyone is trained for this moment and no one needs to be told what to do as it's already being done. In about forty-five seconds from the time the back doors closed, the 7.0 cuffed endotracheal tube is being fed into the messy opening of the airway. The anesthesia specialist somehow just knows were the opening of the trachea is despite the bloody mess to pass the special tube between the vocal chords. It's a total bloody mess so it's an educated guess, despite suctioning as much as possible it's still bad. In no time, the cuff was inflated and the chest started to rise but we noticed it was only the right side of the chest rising.

We soon notice the left chest feels flail with subcutaneous emphysema present from our physical examination. It started to worsen right away with the forced ventilation from the bag valve mask (BVM) now being used. There are diminished sounds of air exchange to the whole left side. We suspected a hemopneumothorax, which explains why the oxygen saturations have always been poor. On most serious traumatic calls, something is always wrong with the airway, the breathing or the circulation that affects the survival of any trauma patient. With everyone trained in Advanced Trauma Life Support (ATLS) the outcomes are greatly improved in all patient care.

The impact was mostly on the driver's side and the left chest wall received the extra trauma from the direct blow. The pelvis, the brain and the left side extremities would most likely have broken but as I was so busy trying to get an airway it wasn't the biggest priority – it will be soon enough. Howie immediately decompresses the left chest wall and we get lots of air out the large bore angiocatheter stuck in the left side of the anterior chest. The physician also gets ready to rapidly insert bilateral chest tubes which is rare in EMS but has proven to save lives right away. I ensured both of the IVs were running well to help reverse the immediate signs and symptoms of hypovolemia. Most often the bad trauma cases will also need some blood transfusions but for now normal saline and TXA will have to do.

The vital signs are improving but the heart rate is up to 135 bpm now which before intubation was 70 which means that a cardiorespiratory arrest was imminent before the airway procedure. That was a close call. I got the Tranexamic Acid (TXA) 1 gm ready in a mini IV bag and started the infusion before the physician even noticed. As I was hanging it he's very impressed with my idea. The STARS crew has two units of blood on board but they elect to initiate them as soon as they get off the ground and give the saline some time to help improve the systemic circulation.

The patient needs fluid resuscitation first of all anyways so the blood products can wait for a little bit. My second IV was ready and I was wise as I used our spare blood tubing as an infusion set and it's flushed with normal saline and ready for the blood products later today. The secondary survey was completed as quickly as possible. The chest tubes are inserted and I noticed both lungs are leaking out excess air and the left chest tube has a considerable amount of blood as the differential diagnosis of a hemopneumothorax was correct. Thank God today the right team was present and this patient has the right interventions before flying. With the right ventilation, the right oxygenation and the correct perfusion, his broken body has a chance to survive this terrible internal assault.

The oral gastric tube is in, the Foley is inserted quickly and the pelvis is bound tightly for transport as we suspect a broken pelvis just on the mechanism of injury (MOI) events. I did not see anything obvious but the trauma team and the radiologist can decide that on arrival at the trauma X-ray room. In a short time, the patient is moved to the waiting air ambulance and they are ready to assume control of our patient. They give us a thumbs-up sign as we back off after he is slid and locked into place in the helicopter. We retreated back to our unit to watch the immediate take off as soon as they have completed the required safety checks. There is no room for error on a takeoff so the pilots get one chance to make it right. Thankfully they always have two pilots in our air ambulance system and errors and tragedy are almost zero, for a very good reason.

Today our real job is done except for the cleaning and restocking of our messy ambulance. Our day is good even if it was a bad day for some other people. It very likely should have been a worse outcome without our divine ALS interventions along with the ground crews, the air crew along with the trauma teams. I was hoping Sarah and her crew had better luck with their patient than we had with ours. It was not something we even thought about until now for we had to much else to think about. Heck, I would never willingly lose my partner, but today it just worked out better to split up as we both had our own patients. The help also split up too, so we divided and we conquered a disaster in the making. Today we tag teamed two critically injured patients with multiple teams very effectively.

Now we needed to drive to the city and rescue my partner or get the other crew to bring her back safe within the next few hours. We made a quick call to deployment and they elected to take us out of service to get our unit back in order. We will just go back to our base with my new temporary crew members, then work on cleaning up the mess and await the return of my real partner. The BLS crew was also taken out of service for a few hours. We have a big mess to clean up and some serious restocking of our units. I realized we have our unit's kits all mixed up which isn't a bad thing but just one more thing to fix when Medic-Three gets back from the city. It was a little bigger mess than I thought.

Overall, the call ended much better than it might have, despite a fatality. It could have been three dead. So, all in all it is better than it could have been. I went and found Ben who is in charge of the scene for the RCMP and he is happy with the outcome. Apparently one drunk driver hit the other car and both vehicles possibly have drunk drivers. Both drivers look to have crossed the centre line. The one dead was ejected from the half ton truck; no one had seat belts on today. There were open beer bottles in both vehicles which tells us everyone injured and the one that was killed was basically from stupidity at its finest moment. Thankfully they never hit someone else. The hard part is one of the police officers will be required to perform notification of the family of the deceased and they will be devastated to find out it was a preventable accident for the most part.

Someday the system needs to change but I'm not holding my breath. Thankfully, they didn't kill an innocent person (if we can call the passenger innocent) but it's not our call or our decision so I don't even think about it anymore. We were released from scene and we grabbed all the extra medical equipment and kits and headed towards our base. Today we are going to get overtime just to clean up a mess. So, all in all it could be worse. Tomorrow starts a new day and as soon as I have a partner, our kits are back in order I will be happy and Sarah will be much happier to be at my side. Hopefully they bring us a fresh Timmy's. "It could happen" and knowing my partner it will happen. Today an extra coffee would just keep me going long enough to get home. Then my golden retrievers could be the responsible adult.

It only took two hours to get our unit cleaned up and my partner was back safe and smiling from ear to ear. I was always amazed how the blood ended up in places it had no right to go. In another thirty minutes, our kits and equipment were checked and our units were ready for the next crew to take over. We had a quick debriefing and overall everyone was happy with the outcome. We all appreciate a good outcome and for all things considered it was still a good day.

We were called into the supervisor's office from the STARS base. The supervisor sat to the side while Sarah and I made ourselves at home for a good chat from the STARS physician. The STARS physician said he would call us back and update us and he kept his word. This physician seemed to be someone special to me for some strange reason. I could not place him or had not remembered seeing him but somehow his voice was all too familiar. It was soothing but indicated someone that was in charge and a someone who was a true leader. This trauma doctor would be someone I could work with again, I was positive.

We were told we were right to bypass the first patient right away as it turns out he ended up in the OR for internal bleeding. Both drivers had blood alcohol levels over the legal limit. The trauma doctor also thanked us for an amazing job and was bugging me for making them look so good with the TXA being in before the patient left the scene, as it was already in the IV mini bag. I told him the best outcome was possible with the perfect team. I also said it's too bad about the deceased patient but I said we never even had a chance to help him. We all knew life deals out fate that way some days. Then the physician surprised me even more. Sometimes you least expect the topic to change. Today it changed and I never even seen this coming. I was speechless. Our paths had crossed before but I could not remember it.

The STARS physician told Sarah and I that he was on the trauma team call when I was brought to the trauma centre after my bad accident. I was now in shock. The physician told us the story from his eyes and what he seen watching the trauma team working so hard on me. He slowly told us the real story. The fact I was unconscious and intubated already made his job much easier so he got to sit back and monitor my airway and keep track of my progress. He was the one who noticed my ICP starting to increase and gave me some mannitol. He ventilated me so carefully to keep my cerebral perfusion as close to perfect as possible. They were very professional that night and the trauma team was extra careful with my every move and with every procedure. They knew Lisa had died and many of them were in tears, all while trying to be professional. They held my hand and told me not to give up when my vital signs were not doing very well in CT and they made sure I had anything and everything that could be done as efficiently as possible. It was all they could do for a fellow EMS staff worker. They too mourned Lisa. They knew we were close and that made their care even more sincere. Unconditional love for our co-workers does exist in people but is much rarer.

They held back the tears as much as possible and they made me as safe as I could be. They even escorted me to the ICU with four extra staff members. They made sure I got extra special care and nothing was spared in my care in the ICU. Thinking back, I never realized I had free TV, a private room and I had a free phone. I didn't really notice but I always had extra flowers that sat in my room. Even when I was too broken or sick to see them they were there. The flowers were on my window ledge and they gave off a healing aroma despite the hospital smells that can be so negative at times. The many staff that was involved in my accident, my immediate care and my post-op care became more involved just because I was considered one of them. They too lost a few nights of sleep knowing they had lost one of their own people. Many lost sleep seeing me broken and many absorbed my pain from my broken heart just from caring so much after the accident.

I never realized the bond the other hospital staff had with the EMS crews was so important or so valuable, even if it was not ever stated. I knew they liked us and they always treated us well but several had a soft spot for our crews. Many in ER had noticed our work and we were respected more than most simply for caring and doing as much as possible for others. We had earned that respect. If Lisa could only see my tears today for the love I had for her. I also had tears for everyone who was on the team that looked after me but also for the crews that dealt with Lisa at the scene of the crash and after the call.

Thinking back the cleanup of our equipment, trauma kits, the medications, and the special drugs and equipment that were all over the highway must have been a nightmare. The broken would have been everywhere and the monitors were smashed. There was nothing left intact. I finally broke down and cried for her. Somehow, I could finally let her go. My EMS family was a lot bigger than I would ever actually really have understood or appreciated. It was now my EMS, my firefighters, my police friends and my hospital family from that day onward.

I didn't realize the effects of the loss of my partner and my injury had directly upset so many of the hospital staff. Sadly, we don't really get to know them as well as we would like as we usually bring them a mess and they assume our disasters. They don't have time to visit or to share their personal stories. They would see us arrive and see our effort into saving lives and they would just assume our role. They see our urgency at triage, the extra work done en route and when we gave report we also many times knew our patients' whole story plus we could tell them where they lived, their family history and if they loved pets in most cases. I would entertain some patients so much I didn't have to use so many narcotics on them. They would get to see my pictures and knew that I had two golden retrievers and they also knew their names but only a few remembered their names.

The hospital staff got to see the many saves even if we don't get to find out the results because the STARS crews many times take over many of our patient disasters. They assumed our saves and they gave us credit even if we never heard it. Ironically, many times the papers noted STARS saved the patients or they were credited for transporting some very sick people from the accidents when it was really a ground crew but that was okay as the patient lived, so it did not matter to us at all.

Over the years, they got some of the highest credit even when our crew or our team did most of the hard work on our arrival. We often would have the patient all packaged up before air transport arrived. If you read the papers it would almost always say STARS saved the lives of the patients involved. If it were not for our care, the interventions by the first responders as well as our quick interventions of others many times the patients would have died. In the end, we know but don't need to say who should get the credit. We didn't care as long as we shared the call; it was fine with us.

So often our extra effort gave the patient a second chance and the STARS crew got the credit for more than they often deserved. But regardless we never cared, as it was still our saves in our hearts and minds. It was too bad they never put our units or our crews on the STARS calendar. The rural services deserved more credit even if they were to humble to share it.

We most like likely used them several hundred times over the years. But the papers don't often tell the truth and say that it was the team effort that saved the patient. It should say the care on scene, as well as the excellent care by the arriving critical care air medical crew helped save a life. It should also give credit to the pilots for flying the patient into the urban center safely for such rapid and immediate care or they would have died. Every part of the system saves lives; it's not just one part.

The benefits of using STARS are subtler but they do exist just the same. If we meet them and they take our patient we go back home. They don't make STARS wait in the hallway for twelve to sixteen hours. Instead of sitting in the hallway we are out doing additional emergency calls so I think it is a cool way to circumvent the inefficient system. So even when STARS took in a less injured patient we were back in service sooner, all in all the system wins.

When we used the system and we utilize or know the shortcuts, the patients ultimately receive better medical care. So, thinking back to our call right now I just know somehow, we are more special or have a role in critical care to others even if they have never spoken about it. I knew after today we often owe the hospital staff an extra amount of appreciation even if at the moment, I wasn't sure what it should be, but it should be something very special. I was so unprepared for this day.

The fact that many of them consider the EMS crews to be one of the family even if many times we don't really think they notice us made me humbler. Today I found out the hospital staff notice more than we gave them credit for. I started to slowly cry again but couldn't say anything. Sarah was sitting beside me and knew something was wrong but she just held my shoulder and looked into my eyes. Today I just realized we mattered to many people even if we never knew their names. The physician from STARS we had worked together even briefly had been a co-worker and that was the way we wanted it to be. But I knew as many had to figure this out in their near future we were all just part of a big EMS and hospital care team.

Our team was bigger and closer than I ever dreamed. After several minutes, I could gradually say a few words so I gave heartfelt thanks to the trauma doctor who, I soon realized, was also crying. He too had seen hell many times. On the day of the accident and today he got to see why he loved to be doing what he did. The team made the difference and nothing could ever take that away from anyone on the team. I humbly told him, "We will see you around, my friend," slowly hung up and gave Sarah an extra-long hug. Then we were out of service for an extra hour sitting and talking to my partner, while our supervisor put a (Do Not Disturb) sign on the office for us both to talk. That's what friends do for friends. It helped me realize even with the shittiest calls you can imagine, good can come out of the waves of any disaster.

Today I learned we all matter, even more than I could imagine. Today we all earned our pay, from the hospital janitor, to the porter and to the tow truck driver who must have had nightmares picking up the pieces after we all drove away. My heart is broken today but it's a good broken. Now it can slowly be put back together. I got the bad out of it and in time my friends, my Pebbles and my Tinsel, can start to rebuild it better and stronger than in the past. More importantly I could let Sarah do her job and I could do mine better. Finally, I could let Lisa go and let her be free to fly the heavens. I started to laugh while crying at the same time knowing that I had two guardian angels again looking after me 24/7. I could not have been more blessed. If you consider my golden retrievers that's four guardian angels

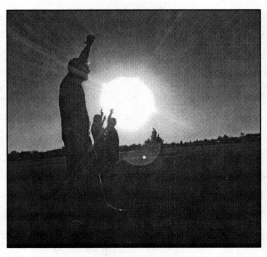

"Standing Strong - Together

"Fighting the Good Fight"

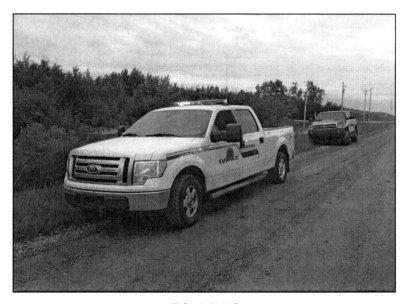

"The RCMP"

"Dedicated to Help us all 24/7"

Chapter Dedication - Special thanks for your dedication. To our RCMP / sheriffs, bylaw, rural and urban community peace officers, as you are always our real-life backup. We thank you for risking your lives and for the dedication of your lives to helping others.

The day started normally with a quick coffee from Timmy's and a little walk with the golden retrievers to keep me from seizing up. I was having a terrible week with pain in all my joints; nothing I tried helped. I was just aching all over. Sarah noticed and had been working extra hard trying to keep me smiling or distracted. She was doing a few extra things for me this week. She could see the pain in my eyes and also saw me taking extra pain medication all tour. She could see and feel my pain. For some reason, this week it's like my joints are all sore and I have no energy to go the extra mile. I had a few bad nights when sleep was not my friend at all. It's all I can do not to cry some nights from the pain. The lack of sleep won't help that out at all.

This tour I just needed to just lie down a few extra times each day to get through them. If I was not doing a call, I was lying down. I think I must have caught a virus as I hurt everywhere. The nights have even been worse on me but I kept going. All I can do is put on some nice quiet music and close my eyes for as long as possible and hang onto my pain. The one song that keeps coming up in my head is amazing. A few lines keep repeating in my head. The song is "Just Be Held" by Casting Crowns. The lyrics "Hold it all together everybody needs you strong," is what I have been trying to do but some days it's not working that well. I'm having more and more trouble being the person that always has it together. Life hits me out of nowhere and takes my breath away. The bad days just come with no warning at any hour of the day and then slowly fade away.

I just wish someone could hold me tight and let me get my life together. I so missed Lisa and others I've lost along the way lately. I thought that they must be the lucky ones. After all, I'm still stuck in this violent and unforgiving world and we must keep going for anything that we are sent to on every call and every shift. I have been trying to lift my head up and keep looking ahead to see a better tomorrow. Even though I'm trying to keep positive thoughts in my head bad ones come along from time to time. I keep having thoughts and bad memories of our past bad or tragic calls suddenly come back. I think they were often some of "life's biggest failures or maybe they are society's errors." We keep having the bad calls and I was sure if someone actually cared about some of our patients we could prevent half of our calls. One study recently said about one-third of the fatal accidents are related to drunk drivers which makes me sick. It would be great if the system could help us have fewer nightmares. People often drink to lessen the pain or take extra pills when they are so ineffective to the original problems. Thus, this all creates more work for us all along with additional death and self destruction.

Today my senses are on hyper alert, expecting bad things to happen at any time. I could not rest or relax. It was almost like being at war but our war is fighting the pain, suffering and our weapons are wisdom along with a few good medications. I was reluctant to over-medicate patients but I didn't want to see people suffering. When we look in the mirror we see the pain with no solution in sight. It's not easy trying to help others when I'm not feeling at my best. I hate being sick but won't call in sick or my partner might have a bad day.

Thankfully my partner was functioning at 120% this week so it's saving me from phoning in sick even if it's justified. I don't want to miss anything and I don't want my partner to work with someone who isn't as nice as I would be to her. I have seen a few staff members treat the EMT staff poorly and two of them are not in our service because of it today. They needed to learn it's a team but they never got it so they went somewhere else to join a second-rate team. Not one person missed them or mourned their loss, but we did help them pack.

Today I was tired of fighting but it's not like I didn't have any other options. Thank God, I had Sarah to keep me together. When I was tired of fighting, tired of being broken and was feeling, so down the answers were further away. As the song says, it's time to just be held. I keep forgetting we are not alone in this world. I think it's a built in self survival technique; even if it's not a good one, it's part of my way of staying alive. My world is not falling apart – it's falling into place. Something I had not quite figured out yet. Here's hoping someone will find me in this storm. When you're on your knees with little hope, someone always comes through, for we are not alone. You can't see the angels beside me but I could feel their presence from time to time. My guardian angel must need to work overtime daily. I actually wondered if they have two of them on me for the nights, but that's stretching resources I would say.

I was thinking about some of most significant staff we have lost over the years today. I then wonder how much longer I have left in this world to do what I do to fight the good fight of helping people. I know about five or six co-workers that have died long before they should have and that breaks my heart even more. We see patients much younger than I am die from strokes, heart attacks and motor vehicle accidents as well as by their own hand all too often. I know I'm not ready to die or to give up just yet. Most days I don't want to kill myself but I feel somewhat pulled towards taking the easy way out. Somehow all the bad calls have a way to bring you down and your days off are just not enough to get you back to being in a better mind space. I sat and thought that mostly the years of terrible events can't be healthy to anyone. Feeling bad about seeing the worst of what the world is our safety net. The day you're not affected is the day you need professional help or you will be forced out of a career in caring for others.

Maybe I'm too sensitive about life, too emotional, too scared or too physically broken and partially worn out but I had to keep going. But being that said I know I can feel pain and suffering and with that I'm still alive. I can see how easily people get lost and missed in this mixed-up and busy world. We need to figure this out a little better, as it's not helpful being a lost soul. We have a coffee date with John, an old friend who is a retired pastor. He will help me out of this deep ditch. I just need to survive a few more shifts. The days off will help me recharge and get some much-needed rest.

The day has been crazy with four calls already and we are still drinking our first coffee of the day. Sarah has my full attention when she announces she going to enrol in Paramedic School right away. I was so happy for her. Her only concern is affording tuition, mortgage payments and being forced to work on her days off to be able to live and afford it. She is eligible for several scholarships but it's not guaranteed. She will apply for them, but she can't count on them. I immediately had a secret plan forming and because I had some extra money in a security safe for education purposes with no real purpose yet, I will ensure she gets supported. I just have to convince her to get her head in the books to study, and the puppies and I will pay her tuition when she is not looking.

I know she has no real family that can help her but I swore to myself she would be looked after, even if she most likely will try to say no. There are ways to help her and we will make it happen. I knew she would do the same for me. I had known since the day we started together, as friends and as partners, I knew she was that right stuff. No matter how it turns out she won't struggle if I can intervene in her life in positive ways.

We are paged out to assist the police on an unknown call. As we pull up, there are no police in sight so I wonder if they are undercover or just not present. The local fire and rescue units are also dispatched but they are not sure what the situation is just yet. They are waiting for an update as well. On arrival, we are staged a block away. There are no updates but we were getting worried as normally we have more information. Today it's an unknown. We have Medic-Three parked on the opposite side of the incident as backup. Fire is also staged, which is very rare. All of a sudden, multiple police vehicle come flying in from different directions and in seconds they have surrounded the house at strategic points. Things just got very serious. We see guns out. They are ready to use lethal force if needed. Nobody is taking chances and they are entering in teams of two to three with each person covering the other. This call just got very real. Today the RCMP were playing for real. Lives were on the line.

In seconds, they make a forced entry in the house from all sides. In another thirty seconds, we are cleared to move in. As we roll up, a tactical member comes to meet us. She tells us they have a young female stabbed in the chest. One other person is in custody. Medic-Three is coming in as well to back us up but it's our patient. The fire members are coming so we have lots of backup. As we walk in we see what looks to be a kid with a central stab wound to the chest with blood everywhere. Looks to be a younger teenager and it looks very bad. We all are shocked to see the amount of blood involved, as the floor is soaked red. Today is going to be a bad day.

As we approach, I take the airway. Sarah assesses the chest and applies an extra dressing. The police have a member already applying direct pressure to the site. The girl is about twelve years old and looks as pale as a ghost. Thankfully Medic-Three is Jim and Tina and they are right behind us. They hurry in and ask, "What do you need?" I simply just say, "About four units of blood and a miracle." Jim applies the LP-15 monitor and Tina punches in an IV. We let dispatch know to launch STARS priority one and ask if they can send a doc and blood as well. I told them we are going to be transporting ASAP and we will be at the local ER in a very short time. We don't give them an option for a scene call, which traditionally is debated. Today there is zero debate. We quickly log roll the patient who has gasping respirations onto the scoop to get her out of here. Dispatch acknowledges STARS is already airborne and have a doc and blood and copy our request. Today we are going to need more than a miracle.

I asked the fire captain to get us a driver and get one of them to bring Medic-Three. We are all going to grab our patient and make a run to the local ER. All hands-on deck. Today it will take everyone and we are still fighting a losing battle but we will fight it at any cost. This kid is going to get a chance, even if life dealt her a losing hand from the very start. Sometimes people have been born into a situation that never gives them a fighting chance – a life of neglect, followed by abuse, and then a lifetime of emotional and physical pain. Of all the calls we hate, these are by far the hardest to do at any time. I can't explain the hopelessness we all feel during or after these calls. Only our eyes tell the story as our words never make it out right.

We have applied high flow nasal prongs at 15-LPM and are ready to bag if the respirations fail. It's only a matter of time I'm sure. We could waste time trying to save a life but it's not going to work. We need a surgical intervention if I'm right. I suspect the knife must have hit the ventricle or ventricles. I'm still not sure how or why she's still alive but she was hanging onto life by a thread. I asked Jim, "Can you intubate her in the unit and then we will take off?" The unit is set up for this type of patient and we have a much more powerful suction; today we need all the help we can get. We need to set up for success and any chance for failure will be availed.

Tina is going to grab our emergency medications we needed right now and prepare them. I will perform a rapid sequence sedation (RSS) but today it's only going to be ketamine as the BP is terrible. This poor kid is so hypotensive we almost won't need medications, which is a terrible sign. She needs to fight a little longer. "We have helping coming, my little girl, you hang on," I told her as loudly as I could. "You fight this, little lady. Don't let go. We've got you." I knew she was in shock but she needed someone on her side.

We were on her team. I don't know who tried to kill her or if we would save her. She can't give up yet, I prayed. Sarah is trying to stop the bleeding but there is blood soaking the dressing. As fast as we applied a dressing, it was soaked again. I looked at Sarah and shook my head "no" to her. We both know where this call is going. We have seen it one too many times. Damn it, why, this is just a kid? Kids should not die this way.

We jumped into the unit and were ready to roll in less than three minutes. The intubation was done and the tube was secured. There is blood everywhere already and the floor is wet and sticky. Everyone is working, doing their best and hardly speaking, as everyone knows what to do without saying it. Jim yells, "A second IV is in" and someone magically grabbed the TXA. I noticed it's also running a little faster than suggested but it's for sure getting infused. We normally don't use it in the paediatric patients but today this is an adult crime and despite our efforts, nothing else is going to help, so why not? We all would say and do it anyways. If someone complains they can complain but their reprimand won't go far. If they were on the call, they would do the same thing, every time, which is all that mattered.

Ben and another tactical member came with us and we were off-scene with a police escort heading to the hospital with police and sheriffs blocking intersections as we went through them without even slowing down. It is a tactical maneuver reserved for only a few situations and this was one of them. An extra officer or firefighter was bringing our back up unit. I never knew who but it came right behind us with siren constantly letting us know we had our backup. We were to busy to care. Unknown to us, the STARS crew is already circling the hospital to get on the landing pad as quickly as possible. We are all totally oblivious to the outside world as we are so busy saving a life. I was just glad the team was working so well together.

Our unit is screaming it's loud siren, which sounds out along with our police escorts'. Time is suddenly in slow motion as we are all working as hard as possible to save a life. We know in our hearts we are the right team today and if there is a chance we will do what it takes. This little lady needs to hold on for just a little longer. I asked someone to quickly patch the ER just as we left the scene so they will be ready. The STARS crew is exiting the helicopter and coming towards the ER as we pull up towards the ER entrance surrounded by police cars, sheriff's' cars, our second unit and a fire truck bringing up the rear. Our convoy made it safely.

A little old man that had seen many things in his years sat on the bench upright and proud and never said a thing. He was a war veteran from two wars and he knew, just as we knew, this must be very bad. In his day, he had seen many tragedies but after hearing about this one, after he got home, he too would weep and mourn as he had for his lost troop mates from wars long ago. Today this call would touch all open hearts.

The Code Blue alarm is already ringing throughout the hospital. We elect to go straight into a trauma room as some days we will just go straight to the landing pad but not today. Today we needed the ER, the ER doctor, as well as the STARS crew and any unused miracle they could find. She won't survive the flight without advanced intervention. As we pull up to the hospital entrance we notice she appears to be going into cardiac arrest. Her heart rate is dropping fast. The C02 is also plummeting which I know means death is coming. The SP02 is not registering anymore as well. But we are not ready to lose this one. We need a miracle and it needs to happen now. We have the right team and if it's possible, life will be pulled out of the hands of the devil. We just need that miracle.

As we were unloading, I could see the ER doc and the STARS crew standing watching as we opened our back doors. I spoke loud and clearly to them in a matter fact voice, "I think we have a lacerated ventricle and we are losing a pulse right now." The two doctors look at each other and yell to the nurses. We then run to the trauma room with our stretcher with our little patient hardly taking up half of the cot. The ER Staff are setting up for an emergency thoracotomy. The physicians are yelling to the charge nurse, "We need more blood as well as fresh frozen plasma if possible. We also need to set up a large bore central line." If there is going to be any chance, this girl will get it today. She is at the right place and we have the right team. We truly were knocking on heavens door with our little lady.

Our STARS doc today is one of my close friends who I have known for years from working with him on many of our serious calls. We all have seen him in action more than once. We know our local ER doc is a gifted emergency and trauma doctor and they are going to team up and do what they can. This just got real serious for the rest of the ER staff about thirty seconds ago, which was just a few seconds before our arrival. In no time, we are in the trauma room. They prepare the chest and in seconds one of them is opening the chest while the second is inserting a big central line. The IVs are running wide open and the blood is coming out faster than we can put it in. We had already given TXA and today it would not slow the bleeding, the hole was just too big to clot off or slow the bleeding down.

The EMS crew and the ER staff are working side by side and as soon as people ask for something to be done, it's done. We are still at the head helping to ventilate this little lady. The doctor asked me to deflate the endotracheal tube cuff and push the tube into the right main stem to ventilate the right lung which we have never done before on purpose. I have seen it migrate into the right mainstem a few times but commonly we ensure the tube is secured so the balloon is in the right spot down a few centimetres in the trachea. In adults, the magic number is 22 cm at the teeth but this is no adult. It's a kid. But today we want the left lung to collapse as the trauma surgeon opens the chest open and we expect the right lung to help keep her ventilated and pray enough blood is circulated with blood to grab some oxygen. Today we needed all the help we could get.

It's just hard to look down and see such a small body with such a terrible hole in the chest. The blood has soaked everything. Our stretcher is now completely saturated in blood. In no time, the ER stretcher was just as bad. I noticed a few extra nurses show up apparently from the OR room but today they might be a little out of their league. This is not a normal procedure for a rural hospital and never will be in my lifetime. But in no time, they step in and assume the roles and the gifted surgeons are thankful, as they need all the help and luck they can get today. The blood is running in wide open, the ER doctor is helping give the blood products and assuming the role of the anesthesiologist and I was demoted which is fine with me. I slowly step back and watch the team in action. Sarah is at my side and she has a hand on my arm holding tight. I then noticed Medic-Three Jim and Tina are standing behind us. We are all watching the gifted surgeons try anything to save this little girl's life.

The surgeon is working on the stab wound and is trying to see where the blood is coming from. It's so much blood the suction can't keep up. He has two suction units suctioning and they can't keep up. In desperation, he clamps the greater vessels feeding the heart and then he sees his worst fear. The end of the ventricle is severed open. He's trying to suture the ventricle but he quickly realizes the futility of the situation and just like that we have lost this horrific battle. Just like that we all simply lost her precious life. One second we had a fighting chance and the next we lost it all.

No matter how good he is as a surgeon, the damage is not repairable especially in this rural setting. If he was in the trauma centre with many more options or had vascular surgical assistance, a bypass pump would have been available but in a rural setting it's not an option. He slowly held his bloody hands up and said. "Stop, we are done." Everyone can tell by his eyes and his voice it's over. In seconds, her little heart was motionless and the respirations simply stopped. Her C02 was not registering and her cardiac monitor was asystole. Our little girl was truly a concrete angel now. Martina McBride would have been so proud of our effort but like her song "Concrete Angel" says near the end of her song so well "but her dreams give her wings and she flies to a place where she is loved, Concrete Angel." Every time I hear the song I think of that little angel.

It didn't seem real, but it was. The blood all over the floor was real. The room smelt of blood and sweat from the heroic effort of people trying their best. The staff was speechless and nothing was said for about thirty seconds. Then the doctor turned to me and my partner. He said, "Guys, we all did a very good job, despite the outcome." He stated the obvious, which was, she should have died in the house but our quick action at least gave her a chance to be saved – if it wasn't for the fact she had no chance no matter what we did. Sarah and Jim said at the same time, "She's just a kid." The tears were running down my face and Sarah wiped them off when she seen them. She too had tears and I wiped them off with the back of my hand.

She got stabbed and is dead from what we call an adult crime but today it's not an adult crime at all. I was still in shock as it looked as though we might have had a chance. We had done everything right. We wasted no time on scene. Despite the delay on arrival, we had no choice but to stage until it was safe. Our care on scene was rapid, transport was rapid, everything that could have been done was done and more. The STARS crew was dispatched early, they had the right doc flying today and the blood they brought was not wasted. Well not directly. It just ran out of the girl faster than it could be put in and that was no one's fault. All in all, everyone lost the battle for a life but not without one great effort. No team had ever worked so hard to save a life. Even though we were all from different teams or groups, everyone molded together to be the right team.

I leaned back and stared ahead, wondering why her? I was wondering how she had stayed alive for as long as she did with such a terrible stab wound but she did. Slowly the staff finish the paperwork and carefully package her up for the trip to the coroner's office because she is now a murder victim. Today this girl has no family to grieve for her. Today we are her family. This doesn't seem right but not one of us would have withheld help even if it were a losing battle right from the start. That's when I started to think about who could have done this and I turned and asked the police the same question. The corporal just shook his head side to side and he too had tears running down his cheek.

It turns out a family member is in custody and is charged with the murder already. Sounds like she is from a house of past hell and the system let another one fall through the cracks. This is why I hate the system as we all too often see it fail over and over. People working in a "politically friendly" world are setting the stage for disaster after disaster. It just seems that all too often people just ignore a bad situation and they commonly say, "it's not my problem" or passing the responsibility to the next person. Someday I hope this is going to change but sadly it's not happening fast enough. Today the system let a girl die. Somehow, we all should be held somewhat responsible for this travesty.

The hospital opened up a staff room to have everyone involved come and debrief. It's an informal debriefing at this time. Hospital staff has arranged coffee and snacks, which arrive for staff that need a break. Even the STARS pilots and police involved were invited in. All too often the public, as well as the professionals, forget that the STARS pilots also see hell over and over on each mission. They too break the limits to save lives but today it was not meant to be. Today everyone lost someone that mattered at least to us. Maybe the rest of the world would not notice her but we would and did our best to save her precious life. Today she was our precious girl even if the world cared less.

Staff mingle and visit while sharing and showing support for every-one involved. No matter what happened they can't take away the EMS, hospital and the medical family effort to save people. No matter what the level of training or their role in the system, today everyone is treated as an equal. After everyone has had a chance to share and reset their emotional clocks, they slowly fade away. After all, Emergency never closes. We walked out to the helicopter with the air medical team and saw them off. We gave them the magic thumbs up as they were ready to initiate their launch sequence. The sound of the rotors changes as they change their pitch and slowly they have lift. It's a strange habit but we always wait and watch them leave and climb over 200 feet before we walk away but today it's even more special. Today we watch them depart and climb and slowly they pick up air speed and in no time, they are several miles out and still climbing.

Nothing else in the world matters right now. My other senses are shut off. My peripheral vision is off. I only hear the sounds of the jet engine burning the Jet A fuel as they depart. I smell the exhaust of the burning fuel in the air as they climb and bank north to return empty to their base. They too are emotionally upset. The pilots, I'm sure, we're looking forward to landing at a trauma hospital and now they are returning minus one soul. The trauma team in the city would be told the outcome and even the dispatchers would have felt the impact of such a tragic event. They remember our urgent calls for days and they too would mourn with us. Many people would be checking on each other in the days to come to ensure the people involved were coping with the tragedy that was likely a preventable death in a perfect world.

I noticed Sarah is at my side and she is in a trance just like me. Today we watched STARS fly away empty without a life being saved. They were leaving us with a bad outcome and we watched them until we couldn't see them anymore. After they were gone I turned to Sarah and gave her a deep hug and then the tears started. The emotional turmoil was released from both of us. The pain and sadness was unbearable; the helplessness we felt watching her bleed out. Then I realized we were both crying. We needed to hold each other and cry. Today we had each other to turn to and life could grant us our time off that we both so needed.

Today we both had someone we trusted and today it was okay to let it go. Today it's okay to simply just say; "This really hurts" Thankfully no one else in the world bothered the two of us, as this was our sacred time. In the distance, the little old man sat in his wheelchair outside with his hat in his hands and he too was crying. He knew our pain despite not knowing our story. He had lost many in the past and everyone mattered to him as well. Today he was our own personal honour guard. We too would also give him our respect every day but especially on May 5th and November 11th of every year. He would always be a soldier and he would always wear a uniform with honour despite his advanced age. He respected us just as much as we too were in a special uniform.

When we finally got our unit back together. I realized, I still had an ePCR to write and we also had Medic-Three, the fire staff, the police and the ER staff to thank as well. I was finally sitting with Sarah doing the ePCR. Sarah stayed with me and made sure I was okay and that I got it done as carefully as we had looked after our patient. We both knew that most likely it might be needed in several years at a murder trial if the legal system even gets the chance.

We were taken out of service for the day. Our supervisor, Greg, called management so an extra crew was brought in. We were paid to be there but we would not be put on another call today for any reason. It was our time to be together with our crews. We got to talk and debrief in our own way. We went to Timmy's, had a coffee and then we sat in the Safeway parking lot and watched the world go past us. Soon we were joined by some of the RCMP on shift. They too made sure we were okay and we were praised for the heroic effort despite the outcome. Medic-Three joined us for a while and we just stayed in the parking lot. They too were taken off from doing emergency calls. We were sharing our personal stories, giving support to each other in our own special way and showed each other we all mattered. Today we had performed a miracle even if we lost the battle for a life. Somehow, we cared more for her in the short time than anyone had in her whole life.

This call taught me that no matter what the outcome, the crews need to work as one. From the RCMP (peace officers, sheriffs), the paid or volunteer firefighters, to the STARS crews and especially the hospital staff, we need to work as one 24/7. At the end of the day no matter if we win or lose we all need to be able to say we did our best. When we work as a team it's much easier to say we did our best when we know it's true. The song that comes to my mind when I'm driving home is exactly the one that is so fitting for today. The song "Concrete Angel" by Martina McBride says it all. It's an amazing song and the video is even better on YouTube. Somehow that video summed up the life of the poor precious girl to a tee.

The part of the song I hear over and over is *"The teachers wonder but she doesn't ask, it's hard to see the pain behind the mask, bearing the burden of a secret storm, sometimes she wishes she was never born."* Then along comes her worst day. Nobody stood at her side to protect her from harm until it was too late. No one intervened until it was too late. No matter how many times intervention could have helped it was not enforced. Nothing is more tragic than child neglect or child abuse, but to see it over and over is pure tragedy.

I can just imagine the pain for the police when they got the call for help from a little girl bleeding and then the line went dead. They swarmed in and took charge. They came to save the little girl. Many of the officers have kids at home and after today's call they go home and love their kids and cry while holding them, but not too tight. Right behind the police came the EMS crews and as the Martina

McBride song could easily have said, *"Through the wind and the rain, they stand as a stone, over and over they fight for the ones that can't fight anymore. In time, she rises above them and watches them work as one but over time as they try everything in vain to save a life she is set free."* Today our little girl got to see we cared for her when the world had turned its back. Today she got to smile looking down from the heavens. Today she was our own concrete angel.

No matter how hard we worked, heaven needs her more than any of us today. Today she earned her wings and maybe the angel of death tried to get her but we brought her back to a safe place. Anyone involved in her care today would have given his or her life for her to live and that's what matters in the end. Sometimes it's all we can do. Today she mattered to strangers and many people showed her she mattered. Then she was free of the pain and free from the hurt. Today she was rescued out of her hell on earth by people who mattered to each other. The final part of the song says it all. *"She stands hard as a stone, in her world she rises above, but in her dream, she is free, she is free from harm and angels give her wings and she flies to where she's loved."*

Through the bad we all must stand and fight for the people who can't fight. In the end the police, the EMS, the firefighters and the hospital staff stood by her side and fought for her life and tried to give her a chance. We made sure no one else could hurt her until heaven was ready to take her home. Then when the time was ready and she was in a safe place, she was set free.

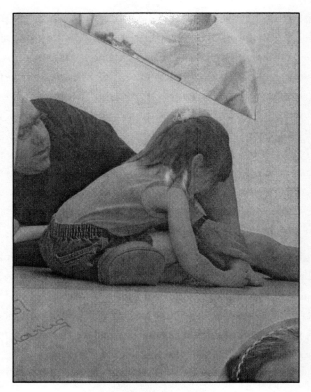

"All Kids Should Matter"

"Knowing When to Walk"

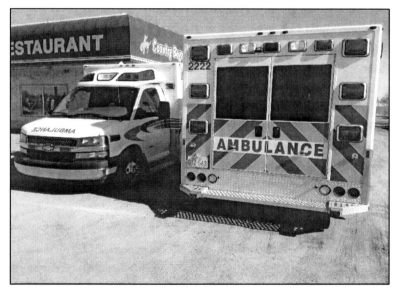

"Saving Lives in Our Mobile Office"

We are called in for some extra relief as they have too many calls. We don't mind. The day has been busy with multiple emergency calls. Sarah is my partner and we grabbed an EMT student for the extra experience who just finished EMT school right after graduation from high school. The supervisor had picked our crew because we were the two best mentors in the service for students. The student, Robin, has a special touch with patients and we are impressed. It is rare to see a student not intimidated by ALS staff, good with patients and wise beyond her years. Most of the calls have been easy today but Robin is right in there on all of them. Even when I was attending she's giving me orders, which I'm not always used to, but they were the right orders just the same. Even Sarah isn't so vocal with me but then I realize Robin is trying to be a leader as a student, which is rare for most students. We just met a lifer for EMS and if we are lucky, she can have my job in a few years.

On the way, we are diverted from coming back home to our base for some much-needed sleep. But the bed has to wait for a sick baby and mother who need our service. On arrival, our student assesses them both and finds they both are unwell. They are not really sick but they both warrant a physician assessment. They both check out okay but then the student thinks they both needed a ride to town for a good reason. As Robin passes me, she quietly whispers to me that this 9-1-1 call is most likely to get them out of a poor home situation. Sometimes we should follow our instincts and our student picked up on it as soon as we walked in the front door. Just with that one important skill I would pass her on a practicum. Robin was gifted as she also had 'spidey sense' already.

It is amazing how Robin picked that up even as a new EMT student. Then I realized she might be more mature for a reason not spoken. Possibly she too had seen a bad home life, despite the actual dispatch reasons. Sometimes we are actually saving or simply helping patients by getting them out of a bad situation. Sarah is attending and Robin is obviously in charge. The transport is going to be unremarkable and I was delegated as the driver tonight, which is okay, as I was tired and Sarah loves to teach. I don't mind driving in the rural areas but not at all in the urban locations. I appreciate it when Sarah is the driver of the unit and I can ignore the busy city traffic. The urban drivers make my BP increase twenty points every time I enter the city limits; it goes down thirty points when we get off the four-lane highway.

The transport is unremarkable until we come across some vehicle crossways on the highway. I automatically think it's a drunk driver at this time of night. I could see a rusty old Chevy suburban across the highway in the middle of nowhere. I activated our emergency lights before I got out of the driver's seat and yelled to Sarah, "Houston we have a problem." We needed to keep other drivers from running into our unit while I was trying an emergency intervention. I was thinking where was the RCMP when we needed them, but I did not have time to call them just yet. I just needed to confirm my suspicion then I would call for police backup.

The driver is slumped over the steering wheel. I had walked up to the other vehicle's door while Sarah and Robin were keeping our patients' safe. As I got to the driver's door I could see the driver is completely intoxicated with a beer in his hand. Then I was sure it's a drunk-driver problem as I called our dispatcher for RCMP backup STAT. They will come as soon as possible but it will take some time just the same. Sometimes things happen for a reason but tonight are one of those nights for me to attempt an intervention. Tonight, I was meant to drive for some reason and this was my moment to stop this man before someone was killed again because of his stupidity. I had seen one too many impaired drivers killing some innocent person.

As I walked up beside the vehicle he somehow must have noticed me or seen our emergency lights flashing and he immediately puts the truck in reverse. This man is driving away from a citizen's arrest. I reached for the door handle as the vehicle started to leave the scene. I couldn't get the door open because he was backing up too fast. Just as I was able to open the door, he just accelerated the vehicle ahead in drive. Pushing the gas pedal down and then the door slammed shut on me. I was racing beside it, running alongside the vehicle and still I couldn't get the door open enough to pull him out of the driver's seat. In seconds, he was out of my reach and he's free to kill someone with a vehicle as a lethal weapon. I was mad at the fact that I almost had him but I was just a second too slow. I called again for police back up and told them the direction of travel. I just hoped that they could now intervene before any tragedy occurred. If it did I would feel partially responsible even if it was not my fault.

I didn't see it but we had RCMP coming from two directions for backup. I didn't really want anyone to know just how close, we had been to stopping him because if he killed someone I would be so upset with myself. I would assume it was my fault for not being fast enough. I then made up my mind this was my battle and I jumped in the driver's seat and decided what the heck, let's stop him. I told them in the back to hang on and we were off. The chase was on. I was going to follow as close as I could and direct the RCMP to stop him or take him out with a spike belt if possible. But in no time, he turned off the highway and took off down a gravel road. After losing too many people there is no way I wanted him to get away. Today I know I was pushing the limits as I had two patients and two staff on board and I couldn't do much more to stop this drunk driver. But suddenly I just knew I must just back off and let the results be as they were to be and I could not continue as it was not our responsibility.

I was praying he wouldn't hit anyone because they wouldn't have a chance against his speeding vehicle. He wouldn't care who he killed and most likely was so drunk he wouldn't even remember driving tonight. He would wake up in twelve to twenty-four hours and deny everything. Then some lawyer would try to blame everyone but the person who was behind the wheel of a 5500-pound human bullet. Believe me, if you're hit by him you're dead. The airbags or the seatbelts can't save you. We can't even save you even though we would die trying if we had too.

Our emergency lights were on and I was hoping he would pull over but today he didn't care. He wasn't about to stop and I didn't know what to do. If I were in a unit with no patients I would have driven faster and stopped him. He's leaving us in the dust. I wasn't sure what to do and all of a sudden, he swerves and hits the ditch and took off into an open field. If I had my own truck the race would have been on and we would have showed him what a real driver could do not impaired. But I could not chase him and my efforts were over before they started. I had already gone too far. I had pushed way past the limits but I couldn't let him kill someone. Not today. Looking back if I could have saved my partner I would have gladly died to save her life. In the end, I did what I had to do despite the risk. Yes, I was wrong which I admitted to Sarah and myself. But sometimes we do the wrong things for the right reasons. This was one of those times.

I pulled over and was about to turn around when I could see his lights going around and around. Now I was mad. I wanted to just go out there and get him, as now he's just teasing me. In no time, the police are coming down the gravel road. I flagged them over and give them directions as to where the vehicle went and they will start the ground search 4x4 style. We took off and headed to the closest hospital. Sarah gave me the look. I looked at her and said I was sorry and meant it. I know she was upset with me for risking myself in the first place when I was running beside the vehicle as she watched me almost get killed or run over. The student was fortunate to miss the crazy stunt but I had to try. I would not feel okay about looking the other way.

We pulled into the hospital bay and the nurses were waiting for us with a smile on their faces as we rolled them into the local emergency room. They were happy to look after the patients especially after we told them about the poor home life we had witnessed. They understood the situation and they will get social services involved in the morning and find them a safer place to live if possible. Just as I was walking out of the emergency room our dispatcher is calling us STAT. I answered them quickly and then I had a smile from ear-to-ear. The dispatcher told me when we had seen the vehicle's lights teasing us it was something we never expected. It was something I could not have predicted. Maybe Karma is on our side tonight. I sure hope so. As long as no one else gets hurt, I'm okay with the outcome.

I had told the dispatcher on the phone line as we drove away from the event earlier on that I thought he was teasing me. I said I would have chased him tonight but I could not due to our circumstances. In reality, when I had seen the lights going around and around, he was rolling over and over. It sounded as though he was spinning in circles and then lost control. Speed and the poor driving ability of an impaired driver is never a good combination. The police say he doesn't look hurt but he was so drunk that he just bounced around inside the rolling vehicle. Thank God, he didn't kill someone else.

In no time, we are running lights and siren down the highway at 140 km/hour and will head back to the gravel road where he had lost us in the dust. Tonight, I pray the deer are off the road and can evade our speeding bullet as several times in the middle of the night I had seen deer on this stretch of the highway. We are at maximum warp as our governor was making our speed limited but safe for our road conditions. The funny thing was that we could see clearly tonight as the dust had settled. The dust would be long gone; the trail would be easy to follow after the RCMP found the fence torn down and the ruts of a vehicle hitting the field at high speed. The chase is over for the RCMP even before they really got started. The lost has been found. Today it would be a simple tow truck driver's problem to bring the vehicle back to the tow yard.

As we pulled onto the gravel road a police suburban flags us down as they have brought us our patient to keep us out of the field. As we get stopped on scene, we are surrounded by police cars and my close RCMP friend is laughing at my story. Quietly he says, "Next time let us chase the bad guys." I acknowledge his reprimand, even if it was more in fun than anything. Sarah and I found the patient handcuffed and passed out in the back of the police truck. Today he's

Between Life & Death

not going to kill anyone. As we assess him, Sarah and the student help scoop him up out of the back of the police truck. He wakes up enough to try and kick the student and then passes out again. Thankfully he missed her and she was expecting it and easily moved out of harm's way.

The cervical collar is applied and he's moved to our unit. Then we realized he's going to be a bigger problem than we expected. I suspected it's alcohol poisoning but we can't take the chance. We suspect he will be okay but then he might be very intoxicated to the point he can obstruct his own airway. It also could be a significant head injury or both problems. He also could have been assaulted before the crash – as I didn't get a good look at him and that could also be a very likely possibility. We elect to intubate him and over time they can figure it out in the city. At least he's not driving down the highway and no one will die from this drunk driver tonight.

It was amazing how someone's day, such as our patients, started out and how it would end intubated waking up in a city hospital with no license and no vehicle. I bet this morning before his first drink he would have never imagined waking up in the emergency room or after a short ICU stay. Most likely all he really needed was a basic trauma panel lab test, a quick CT scan and a few X-rays. We know from many repeated calls that; the drunk drivers are not usually injured. I keep asking myself why do people drink and drive? I will never know the answer to that one single question.

So, all-in-all it could be worse for me and thankfully for him we can ensure he doesn't die from either problem. Thank God, he never killed someone and only hurt himself. I think to myself, "sometimes we win and sometimes we lose". Sarah is setting up the intubation equipment and helping the EMT student ventilate and apply the cardiac monitor, SpO2 is 100%. The end tidal CO2 is thirty-seven mmHg, that is okay for now as the range is 35-40 for a head injury patient. We have two good IVs established already. Our first vital

163

signs are good. The heart rate is 118 bpm. The respirations are 12 and shallow but it's adequate. The BP is 145/94 so I elected to give Versed® 5 mg and Fentanyl® 200 mcg IV as he's a larger person and all the vital signs are stable. I elected to administer the Anectine® 120 mg as it's drawn up and ready. I don't want to fight with this airway and it's sometimes better to properly medicate at a higher dose to get the airway the first time. I was never one to miss a tube if it was at all possible. Plan for success was the golden rule.

I put the laryngoscope in and I can see the vocal chords easily. I passed the endotracheal tube easily. The vocal chords were actually waiting for my tube so it was easier than expected but most likely a benefit of the appropriate medications prior to our attempt. I confirmed the placement and the CO_2 is good at 35 mmHg now. The SpO_2 is 100% still so we are okay. Our local dispatcher notified us that STARS must have been delayed launching and elected to meet us at the local ER helicopter landing pad instead of the scene, which was fine with us. The police are happy to escort us to the local landing pad, which is right beside our most favourite ER in the world.

We transported to the local helicopter pad without incident. We were required to add more sedation en route but that's easy to accommodate. The aircrew took over and the RCMP officer was more than happy to be an escort for us and for the fight, as he will get a free ride out of this night as well and that's a cool night. He will be going with the patient to ensure he gets charged with impaired driving correctly and that the blood sample meets the legal requirements. Maybe, just maybe, one drunk driver will be off the road, for a little while at least. It could help save at least one life if the system keeps him off the road.

Overall, the call went not too bad, despite how it started. Sarah and Robin told me afterwards they were happy to have such a good outcome. Thinking back, it could have been bad if I'd got run over at the start of the call. It could easily have happened. No matter how we plan our call or think our day will unfold, things will just happen. After the helicopter had gone I was still writing the ePCR for a little while and not really paying attention to anything until I noticed Robin sit down beside me. I was actually shocked or maybe a little surprised because she looked worried or perplexed. I thought maybe I had done something wrong. After all, I had made a few unwise choices tonight. They could easily be justified in being upset with me after our crazy ride. I asked her what's up with sincerity. "I wanted to talk to you about my future," she said. "I need to know I'm making the right career choice but sometimes I'm not sure". I finished my ePCR and said, "Let's talk." I have all the time in the world right now for her. Robin deserves my full attention and she will get it. I know looking into her eyes she is one of the most caring people I had ever met other than Sarah.

Robin asked me one hard question right off the start. The question was simply, "Was it worth it?" I knew exactly what she was thinking or asking me right then. I have asked myself the same question a thousand times over my whole career. I told her that I asked myself the same question to myself over a thousand times as well. Sometimes I wasn't sure at the time but tonight I had an answer. Somehow, I had figured it out in my mind but could not or had not shared it with anyone else as of yet. I thought about my response and then I said it just like I had thought about it.

I said for the ability to help people, it was worth it. It has its many rewards that are not money. It also has some bad times as well. Yes, it was worth every damn broken heart. It was worth every nightmare, it was worth the sleepless days and the long stressful nights. It was even worth it tonight, to try and stop that drunk from driving, even if it almost got me hurt in the process. Mostly I do it for fun in my mind, I have never considered it a job. Then at the end of the day or the end of my tour, it's over and what happened is past. What happens next tour is in the future.

I can't add the ones I saved or helped. I carefully tracked the ones I lost and for a good reason. I learned from every patient I ever had. Even if the lessons were unfair or harder than others. Living should count for everyone but dying also should count for something as well. Robyn just sat and listened, after I had finished, she looked out of the backup unit. I gave her time to ponder my answer.

Then Robin asked me, "Do you think I could be a paramedic?" She looked into my eyes and said, "I don't know if I have what it takes. Just last night I saw many things they don't teach us in school." I had to think of the response. I told her:

"School is just a start in your formal basic EMS education." Sometimes the best knowledge or best education in our EMS field comes from the roads of life that we are travelling. The education from the life we live, helping others is the best but often hardest. Life's lessons are sometimes hard, and often unforgiving. When it comes to human life, regardless, they are still lessons. Yes, sometimes I don't know what to do and you will always come across things or calls you have never seen in the past. That's why you have a partner. We are part of a team. That's why we have backup. We can always call someone and ask, so it's not like we need to know or can know everything because that's impossible.

Even the best trauma doctor will have some wisdom that's not in his book of tricks. Somehow, we all just simply figure certain problems out. That's why it's a lifelong learning event. "Robin, as an EMT, you will help others and yes, we save lives but as a paramedic you go to the next level. The more we learn the bigger the challenges are. The harder the challenges are, the more interventions we need to master. It's like checkers, a starting point in life, finishing a game of chess and winning almost every time. The most logical reason to be a paramedic is to save lives. We can make a difference as long as we always give 110%. Anything less and it won't work."

"I've seen many people start out with high hopes and big dreams but over the years they eventually gave just a little less towards their job – now they are not working in the industry anymore. If you want to be a paramedic you need to make the commitment or don't walk down this road. I've made a difference for thousands. I have helped even more, as well as I have made many more people have a better day, than you could ever imagine. There is nothing like talking to someone a few days after they had a cardiac arrest. The sure way to help others is simply to care more and more. The more we care, the more we can help others." But the caring comes with a personal cost that we need to be able to bear.

Then Robin surprised me with a simple but appropriate question. "But doesn't it give you pain or nightmares after some of our bad calls?" I thought about this even longer. My answer is not as easy as the rest had been. But it's not that hard to admit to someone I trusted. Today I made a new friend and Robin is someone I now trust with my life, my fears and my inner-most secrets. So, I could tell her my secrets and my pain. I could share with her some of the biggest mistakes in my career in the hope she would not make the same mistake. Life's lesson can be shared with our friends. By sharing my past mistakes, I was sharing my wisdom. With wisdom comes knowledge and with knowledge comes better wisdom.

I looked into her eyes with honesty and sincerity. My words were from my heart. "Well I guess it's the cost of the job. No job is perfect. We don't have a perfect world. We don't live in a perfect world you might say." I thought about it some more and then I told her my real feelings. "The ones that hurt me more are the ones that should have lived but we could not save them. They were the ones that shouldn't have died - the innocent ones. I think back to last night's case, for example. The drunks are killing the innocent and our system allows it to happen over and over. Then we have the senseless critical stabbings and the even more senseless murders. We have more and more school or gang-related shootings. I thought back to the police who had been stalked and shot over the years at Mayerthorpe, Moncton, St. Albert and the other places that still haunt our sleep from time to time." It still seems unreal. All we can hope to do is change the ones we can touch.

Robin asked me a really good final question. Robin asked the question "How do we change our EMS profession for our future co-workers?" It made me think a bit about her question. Then I shared my thoughts. "Robyn, over the last several years, I've been looking ahead towards our future in EMS and we have lots of positive benefits to look forward to in some areas but not in everything". Looking back, we needed the change but I challenged many to see it with their own eyes. Sadly, we are in trouble as a profession – if we don't excel in everything we do, we will fail. We need to push the current limits of our paramedic practice and exceed the minimum of the current standards in the EMS education world. We need to create new EMS members to be the leaders in the healthcare world as well.

Robin, I don't know if the current EMS culture is ready and willing to make the positive changes needed. The biggest reason is people don't like change because it takes effort and not all change is easy. I wonder most days if we are going to get stuck in a rut with slow progress where we keep changing gears but not going ahead. It's like walking ahead one step but then needing to go back two steps every time we get ahead. It's not very reassuring to the public if we are not trying to excel but be followers in the healthcare system. We need to lead the profession and at the same time we need to be an equal member in health care and not someone's aide or servant.

We can't just sit back and see the world go past without some good intervention being applied and some extra effort being made for a positive change because doing it the easy way won't make it better in the end. We can't promote negative communication but we won't ignore the negative feedback from an industry that is frustrated by the lack of influential good leadership. Somehow or someway, we need to get up and build our profession from the ground up.

Think back to school and remember the student that complained the loudest about the extra reading or the extra assignments. They were the ones saying they felt this was a complete waste of time and effort. That is the world we are in right now. The negative concerns are something we must deal with to ensure it doesn't weaken or put our profession down. We must not walk a pathway in life that reinforces negativity. We need to turn our whole profession towards being in the positive. We need a positive outlook for all of our members within our profession to be successful. We need to build our profession as a positive and a stronger team.

We must be able to turn around when we head down a bad road or hit a dead end in our lives. Then we need to start going down the right road for the right reasons. I love the saying from Joe from the Movie Unconditional. Joe states "It's not a dead end if it takes you somewhere you needed to go." Some of the roads we travel down will be wide open roads and it will be easy. But along the way we must climb a few hills that will enhance or elevate the EMS profession as a whole. We must prove to our allied health care members that we deserve to be the leaders of our profession.

Our EMS world needs us to function at an optimal level, despite the limitations imposed on us by the current level of care or our current protocols. If we continue to be followers in health care, we will lose our true identity. If we don't fix our weak and broken system and make some global changes, we are doomed before we even start. It's time for people to stand up and be proud of who and what we are as a professional body. We need to make an EMS system that is second to none. Let's be winners. Let's work for a unified change to be the members people count on 24/7. Robin, this fight is not mine anymore but you and people like Sarah are the ones who need to strive to care enough and show your vision of the future to others in our profession. We must become the leaders of our profession over time.

"Recently, I lost my partner and I guess it made me realize even more that life has no guarantee of tomorrow. People keep saying tomorrow they can do something important such as call a loved one or take time to have coffee with a special friend, or plan a trip to see family but many don't take the time. You need to spend time with your loved ones. Tomorrow is never guaranteed. The right now, is all we get for sure. It's what we do with today and right now that counts for our tomorrow, my friend."

Out of the corner of my eye I now could see that Sarah was standing there just listening. She was thinking about what I had said about the profession. Especially the negative people that have been in her life and how since she was partnered with me, one big problem went away. Her last partner was always negative and when the tones went off, the complaining started. That is why after being an EMT she left the rural service where she started at and moved on. Looking back, she chose the right options. I would not have made it without her – and she made our team the real winning team. Even though she was an EMT she was miles ahead of me in many things and that was what counted to us as a team. Without each other we would not have made our successes possible. With the worst team effort, the results are predictable. With the right people, the success stories are also possible.

I turned to look at her and notice she is crying but smiling at the same time. I smiled back and nodded my head to her. We had just the right partners tonight and that made us have the right stuff. I turned to Robin and said earnestly, "Now get your application done for the provincial exam and after a little life experience you get into a good paramedic school so I can retire. When you're ready, let me know and I will give you a reference. I can help you get a few books that you will need. I have a good friend going to school very soon and she might have a few books as well." Sarah just smiled at me and she got my message loud and crystal clear.

I looked at Robin and told her, "Heck I'm too damn old for this job anymore, so you'd better get it done sooner rather than later." I smiled as I looked right at her. She walked over and gave me a big hug and then turned and gave Sarah an even bigger hug and thanked us both for such a great night. Tonight, I showed a new EMS member what it's like to have people to count on. We were a family of people who mattered and she was special so she mattered even more. No matter what she needed from that day on we would ensure she got through her challenges and in time she would be on our team. I was sure of it.

I had my ePCR done and it was time for a little sleep if at all possible. At least I could try my best to lay down and take what I could get. After all, a few minutes is sometimes better than none. I would almost kill for at least ten minutes of sleep right about now. I needed it just long enough to close my eyes and relax. Thankfully we only had four hours left on our extra shift and then I was on days off. These days off I was taking for myself. I'm planning on taking my goldens for a drive and will spoil them rotten. I have a few good friends on shift on a nearby service, Kevin and Clarrisa, and I'm going to surprise them both with coffee. I just need to survive a few more hours myself.

In the morning, I said goodbye to Robin and we exchanged numbers and emails. I shared with her some contact information for good schools and made sure she was aware she needed to get going on her applications ASAP. Sarah also made sure she was on the right track. We decided to go to Smitty's after work and had a great breakfast together; the goldens got to meet Robin after our breakfast. They just adored her like she was part of the family. They even found some of the bacon I saved for them in a napkin from my pocket. We said goodbye in the parking lot and I smiled as I watched them walk away as a team planning their next visit which I was sure would be really soon.

I sat in my truck and thought about a very bad day in my past, which had changed my life forever. It was the day one of our co-workers lost her spouse in a very sad and tragic way. It was a day right out of hell. You could not have experienced a worse event but looking back it brought many of us closer together. So, all in all life happens for a reason but we often don't know the reason at the time. Robin was meant to come to be our student just as we were meant to be her mentor for the start of her EMS life.

As I sat and just thought about life I realized that there comes a time when I had to stand up and fight our system but I was not sure I had one more fight in me. We need to stand up for our EMS family members. I have seen others look away from those in trouble but that is not in my creed. We are a band of brothers and sisters 24/7. This may mean at work, on a call, after the call and after we go home. Sometimes we know our partners are in trouble but we tend to want for them to ask for help or to say it's not really my problem.

Yes, some days we want to give them their space and respect their right for privacy but we know the calls we see can be so traumatic for others. It's not just one call usually, it's the calls, the types of call, or possibly the situations around the call that affect us all so differently. My biggest ones are the sick or dying kids. But when it came to see one of my friends and co-worker on her worst day, nothing else in the whole world could top some of those very bad days.

After many years, they are the ones that are the hardest to let go. My biggest and hardest day was coming to work when my good friend's husband shot himself. Some days you can take it and it doesn't bother me but that day I will not forget. Not many of us will. Some things are ingrained in a part of our brain to prove we are really human, or maybe too human I would have to say. Well I was never going to expect this day to occur but I should have known that even worse things were yet to come. Sometimes the world sends us messages that bad things are coming right at us.

I was coming to work early one day; a rare day shift as I hate day shifts. Just as I topped the Gwynne Hill I was listening to the song from Matt Anderson and I was not paying much attention. Just then the words struck me very clearly. The song was "When my Angel gets the Blues." *"Little girl. I'll follow you down, I don't care how far we go, I need to see you get your feet back on the ground, you don't need to tell me, 'cause I don't need to know, it hurts so bad, every time she cries, when I was there to wipe the tears from her eyes, it hurts so bad. Every time she cries"* – the meaning was so clear to me. As I walked into work I met my friends and they told me the bad news. I went into the trauma room and there she was. I have never seen anyone so broken, so hurt, so needing us all in my whole life. I still could not and will never understand how someone with so much heart, so caring of a person, could be put through this hell.

I still don't know why it hit me so hard that day. The look in her eyes was more pain and more hurt than I had seen in a lifetime of bad times. I did not know what to say. Many of the people there had been my friends and co-workers for years. That day showed me we need to be able to stand beside our hurt co-workers. We don't need to say anything but we need to stand together. I knew that day we all needed to do more to help our friends and our co-workers before, during and after a traumatic event. We see death and destruction every day but when it's one of our own family members involved it hurts that much more. Today we were all a family and we stood our ground for each other.

I know that day was so traumatic for the ER staff and the paramedics that knew her or had worked with her for years. We all wanted to help and there was nothing we could do but try our best. Thankfully she had such loyal and dedicated friends she was never left alone. To know people thought the world of her must have helped her through the darkest days that were to come along. That day taught me it is okay to not be okay or to cry. To this day and for the rest of my life I hope I never see that much pain in anyone's eyes, especially from someone I consider my friend.

In the end, it was a good tour. Now it was time to sleep. Later I had to get up and see my family doctor. I was sure he would give me some good advice. Even if I was not happy about it I would do as he suggested. Sleep came easily for me that day and when I woke up with my golden retrievers bugging me. I felt I had been asleep for a day but in reality, it was only four hours. It was as good as I expected and soon we were off on another adventure. The day still had some good things to show me and I needed all I could get, so off we went.

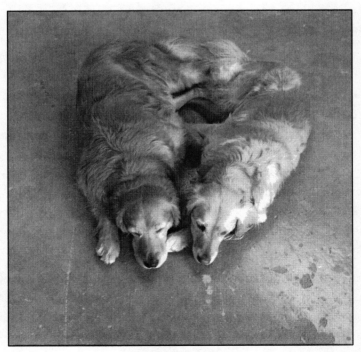

"Love Knows No Limits"

"Family Friends First"

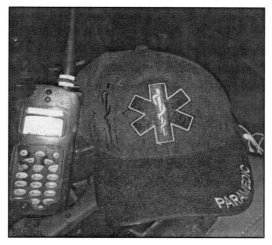

"Even We Can Lose our Perspective in Life from Time to Time"

Sometimes in our EMS profession and in health care we need a life break. Nothing is more therapeutic than packing up and going somewhere special for a good reason. I currently had nothing planned this week other than staying on my back deck, thinking about life and staying alive. Maybe I would have a few drinks or a few beers (*most likely a root beer float would make my day*) but all in all it's still beer. Then I would do some yard work. Somehow, I was going to be able to slow down and watch my life go past in slow motion. I needed to reset my life and this was one way to stop and get back on track. It was much better than being locked in a padded room where I'd seen a few of my co-workers end up over the years. Sadly, once you are broken that badly you can never ever come back to the same. It was almost like being struck by lightning, it was a life-changing event if you lived. The keyword was the "if." I would have to say.

I had an unplanned month off on my doctor's recommendation and he asked me to see a psychologist trained in PTSD as well. I had been down in the dumps with just a little too much badness built up inside for a lifetime. I had never seen anyone in the past; it would be a new step. It scared the life out of me but I had promised my friend I would go. I kept my promises. Even though my last week was great, the week before was not so good. I was going to be seeing a counsellor for PTSD but it was taking time to get in and be seen regularly. Now that I was off I thought I could do some personal rebuilding for myself. I had no real desire to go anywhere special or do anything. I most likely was depressed or just beyond being sad. I just wished I had somewhere to go, someone to bug but nothing had come to mind yet. I needed a pick-me-up but was not ready to call anyone because it would seem too strange. Many of the events we have seen over the years we don't want to share with most people other than someone in our field of care. It would have to be someone in healthcare, a police officer, a firefighter or only a select few friends that I trusted. That was whom I trusted the most with my life 24/7 already. I had no reason not to trust them. They would and could understand my inner pain and suffering. I had no choice too, as they were my real family.

One of my therapeutic goals this month was to come up with a better outlet for stress relief. Many don't realize that it doesn't show on the outside but builds up on the inside, much like an evil disease. I had really wanted to spend time with some personal friends and get time to work on my ability to describe my worst days to a person or small group of people I trusted, such as a PTSD support group. So far, the meetings did not work with my schedule. You just know your life is too busy to schedule a much-needed massage therapy session.

We all have many friends around the world that I would love to see but they must be busy and I don't want to intrude in others' lives. Most are always too busy to just drop everything and visit with me for a few days. But I thought sometimes friends can always use some help from time to time and I'd love a working holiday. Many people might think I was nuts but it's my kind of a holiday. Sometimes our friends need us. We are only a call away but they don't call because they think we are also too busy. The way it's going, however, even my golden retrievers will get bored with me. It's not happened yet but it's heading that way. I have had a bad year so this break needs to be a long one and I have a month off. That's not my idea but my boss and my doctor said it's time for a break. Seeing death, pain, suffering, with repeated exposures to badness must take a toll on everyone including Superman. So, it was time to recharge away from the evil forces of nature or away from the EMS world I would say.

Out of the blue I was sitting on the back deck watching the planes land and take off from the local airport and I got a strange call at just after 06:00 a.m. It's early for a long-distance call and it made me think the worst. The call was from a 306-area code, which is Saskatchewan, my home province, and the number is familiar but not called in several years. It's from a family friend I haven't seen for several years.

As soon as I answered I knew it was Don. Don was one of my classmates from elementary school and a family friend I have kept in touch with over the years but not often enough. Our life schedules and the distance have kept us apart but our friendship has never changed. Even if we can't see each other very often we simply pick up our conversation where we left off. Don is a farmer and has been farming on his own for almost fifteen years now. Don had taken over his dad's farm and has been a hard worker all his life. He was calling to see if there was any way I could come and help him for a bit as he needs a volunteer even if it is just for a week.

Don says he has a lot of hay to be taken off and it's ready to cut. He has a bunch of other things that have needed to be done but life had not let him get caught up recently. This year he's run into a big problem. He had been working long hours and got a nasty laceration that was now infected from a metal sliver in a work-related incident. It didn't heal very well and now he's got a swollen leg, unable to work for a few weeks. The doctors had found the dirty metal sliver and removed it but it will take time to heal. He's going to be getting IV antibiotics for at least two weeks and for a farmer, that doesn't work at all. He needs to farm and to be at the local hospital two or three times a day for a double therapy of antibiotics is not going to help.

With the infection in one leg and in no time, he's too sick to walk, let alone work long hours. His doctor wants him off his leg and on the couch or in the house for two weeks. That is almost impossible at this time of year for any farmer. He was not sure what to do as he's got no family left nearby and good help is hard to find anymore. Nobody wants to farm it seems. It's hard work for not much pay, long hours and it takes multiple skills.

So out of the blue he remembered when we were kids that I loved to farm, took a chance and called me up. I needed a break and this call came at the right time. It's strange but sometimes life happens for a reason, even if we don't understand, it still occurs. His wife is an angel but she's not much into driving farm animals and she has three little girls to keep out of trouble so her days are even busier now, looking after her husband.

The last time we met we had supper in town with them about two years ago. They were on their way to the West Edmonton Mall and stopped for a short but a good visit. I told them both, if they ever needed anything, just call. Over the years, we have stayed at their place and they have stayed at my place as well. Well, Don called and I can tell he is down. With no family to back him up he needs me, even if he's a little embarrassed to ask. I know he's very strong, hardworking, a great father, husband and a very honest, proud man but sometimes we hit a wall and things get us down. I can hear that in his voice. I know he would not have called unless he needed help and today he needs my help. I was not about to say anything but yes.

Everyone that is human and normal will have bad times in life. Sometimes people need to be rescued and we just have to drop what we are doing to help them before it's too late. I never hesitated and in a second I had a solution to his problem. I shared with him my problems and we made a pact to help each other. My reward might be paid in frozen beef in my freezer after we came home but it was still worth it and we got a holiday having fun. He would get some good honest help in exchange for my therapeutic break from a crazy stressful EMS life. My bad times would slowly go away with some fresh air and the freedom of the outdoors. His misfortune would go away with rest and antibiotics. It was a win-win for us both in the end.

I never even thought twice about saying no. I needed something special and in no time, it was provided to me. I was getting "divine intervention" right from a higher power and Don was getting someone to help him out, the same way. I thought maybe our guardian angels were cousins, but then that is too deep a thought this early in the morning. It was time to drink my coffee and get going for the day. It was going to be a busy one.

It's strange that I was worried about trying to find something that appealed to me for my therapy. I needed some physical labour and I wanted sunlight for a change. Sometimes our prayers are answered even if no one heard them but our guardian angels and maybe God. But a miracle just helped my messed-up world get better with one phone call. So, in no time I had the perfect solution. They need someone they trusted to help them and they are in big trouble. After a ten minute phone call, I could understand Don's needs and it was simple. He needed someone special who could work independently and do whatever needed to be done on the farm. Thankfully I was raised on a farm and never stopped learning, so when it comes to fixing, building or looking after people or animals I've got it figured out and I was able to jump on any tractor. So, this is a therapeutic holiday in the making already.

The strangest thing was he called when I was in need of therapy. I was put off work on a four week doctor ordered holiday for medical reasons. I needed some time away from the evil world. I had nothing planned, as it was not a scheduled holiday. It was to get my mind and body healthy or I would get locked up, I thought. In fact, I was going to be bored stupid and didn't have any projects booked other than a weekly session with a good therapist. That wasn't something I looked forward to but it was required to stay well mentally.

I knew I could not sit doing nothing but I also knew I would need a project or something to build to keep me sane. I was trying to think up a project but nothing made me very excited until this call came along. I will call the therapist in a few hours. In no time, I will be receiving a therapeutic session even if it's while the cruise control was set at 103 km/hour. I could not think of a better therapeutic session than driving a tractor, watching the field go past me in real time.

After talking to Don, I realized that they had had a few bad years with farming and at least two bad years of crop failures that have hurt everyone in the whole region. Between the extra rain, then flooding and the drought, they just can't seem to win. They run a mixed farm with crops, hay and beef cattle. They worked hard building their farm up from nothing but then nature doesn't let us get away without having some bad times along with the good times.

Don and his wife Sally will be waiting for me in twenty-four hours and they will show me pure love and respect from the bottom of their hearts. They have three little ladies that would love to see my golden retrievers even more than me, most likely. They have Josie who is eight, followed by Memory who is four and Aimee who is two and a half. I'm sure they are going to be very happy to meet Pebbles and Tinsel. In no time, they will be spending time with my golden retrievers. They just lost Jack, the family dog that protected them until one night recently when some predator or predators lured him away from the house. Don found him when it was too late. So, Pebbles and Tinsel might fill that void until they can afford a new farm dog I thought as I packed my bags for a working vacation.

I simply said, "I'm packing my bags and we'll see you tomorrow for breakfast." I asked him if he'd have a problem with a few extra mouths to feed. Most people have a farm dog; sadly, they'd just lost Jack. But he assured me it's more than okay to bring my two extra passengers. I knew they too would more than love a farming holiday, instead of being cooped up with me at home. They just happen to have a fifth wheel that can be parked just across in an open old farmyard by an old barn. There are grain bins and a modern shop in the yard as well. It has power and water to the yard site so life will be pretty easy for me. It will be like camping but in a modern world with no pagers or radios.

In two hours, I was packed. The golden retrievers got in the truck about an hour before I was ready to go. Pebbles is keeping the backseat warm and is stretched out sleeping. Tinsel is sitting up front watching me pack with a very careful set of eyes. There was no way they would take a chance on missing this trip. They know we are going but have no idea it's a real outdoor holiday. We even packed a few extra things that I don't ever get to use on my mountain holidays, but on a big open farm with predators it's a little different. I packed a few good rifles and my dependable 338 Winchester Magnum with the three-round clip. I also took ten extra rounds as this is about all my shoulder can handle, and my old 30/30 for the really small rodents. With my 338 Winchester Magnum, if I can see a predator,

I can reach out and make them a non-predator. Just maybe we can look after Jack's killers the right way. An eye for an eye they say is the right way in the country.

For the next several weeks, I won't need a portable radio or a pager and that will be a blessing. My trusty iPhone was my alarm clock, my music player and the only way to communicate with the people I want to reach out and visit with from time to time. Most often it's people calling me for advice and that's okay as well. As soon as we hit the highway the cruise control was set to the speed limit plus three just for good measure. My Red Dodge 1500 (Ramone2) has an Eco-diesel 3.0 and for some crazy reason that's where we get the best fuel economy. Pebbles and Tinsel were curled up on the back seat enjoying my audiobook while they slept.

I have an audio book playing and for the next twelve hours we are going to be chasing the world of bad guys. This trip, John Clarke is eliminating some drug dealers while helping the CIA rescue prisoners of war in Tom Clancy's *Without Remorse*. We only need to stop for fuel one time and stops on the rest of the trip are solely to make the puppies comfortable. They have food and water so they don't need anything but bathroom breaks. We stop whenever they look funny – that is the message it's time to find a bathroom. I will get a few cups of coffee along the way to keep my eyes open. The road is mine and after the sun goes down I need to turn on my special senses to make sure I don't hit a deer or a drunk driver doesn't revoke my birth certificate.

The drive was uneventful in Ramone2. I still miss my F250 Ford Diesel 4x4 but a moose decided to kill it for me one night just out of Sherwood Park. Sadly, it wasn't even moose season so we never got to tag it but my truck sure did. In a heartbeat, it was broken beyond repair. That truck was the toughest and most loyal 4x4 I had ever had and with a snow plow mounted on the front, we made any snow road a possibility. Now my new truck Ramone2 would have to take over the challenge and it too would need to keep my puppies and me safe. We had a long way to go and eighteen hours to get there.

The trip went well with no drunks or crazy drivers trying to kill me. Still it's a 1000 km trip so with breaks and puppy stops it's normally a thirteen-hour trip. But as we promised, we had a little sleep before arriving and we pulled up at 06:30 just in time for some breakfast. Heck life isn't so bad with a breakfast of champions – we have steak and eggs waiting for us.

Slowly some happy faces come out of their bedrooms and smile at me as they peek at me from around the corner in the kitchen. That is until they see my puppies lying by the front door and then they are all over them. Pebbles and Tinsel are now show-and-tell items for all the girls and they are quickly shown around the house. The puppies get equal portions and everyone is on holiday and being treated like kings. After being there for ten minutes it was just like we left our last visit. It's amazing how friends can pick up right where they left off. Both the goldens have tails wagging so hard they almost knock over little Aimee but she doesn't object.

It just shows me that love can exist everywhere and all it takes is an open heart. In no time, Pebbles and Tinsel are making the little angels feel as though they are in heaven. They are smiling and hugging the puppies and secretly giving them extra breakfast snacks off their plates. As I head out to work the girls are fighting over who gets to sleep with the puppies tonight. Three girls with two puppies, I might have to sleep alone but I'm 110% okay with that. The girls will put Pebbles and Tinsel to work being guard dogs I'm sure and that is important right now.

Over breakfast Don told me the sad news about Jack. He had searched and found Jack, right after he took off after something out in the barnyard. When Don found him, he could tell he put up a good fight but it was too darn late and the killers were long gone. Don told me he thinks it looks like a pack of wild dogs. He didn't see them but heard the vicious fight in the middle of the night. Jack was doing his job protecting his people and gave his life up for them. He went everywhere outside with the girls. He never left them unattended when they were outside. He must have known killers were around. That dedication cost him his life but he was rewarded with their love.

Thinking aloud, Don says coyotes normally kill around sunrise but it's hard to tell. They live along a river so it could be a cougar as they are around, but rare. If Pebbles the Wolf had been around she would have turned the tide and with Tinsel the Terminator at her side they would have given Jack some really good backup. But for the next few weeks we can make the family just a little safer if the killers come back. I won't go anywhere without my rifles so Jack's loss will be avenged if I get a chance. I just need that one chance and my 338 will do the rest. I could not miss the opportunity to avenge the loss of poor Jack.

After breakfast is done we have already figured out a plan of attack to get some farming done. In no time, I have the next week's worth of work planned. In an hour, I was out in yard with the 2290 Case pulling a fifteen-foot New Holland HAYBINE® Mower-Conditioner. It is amazing – I haven't used one for about ten years and it's like I just used it last week. The HAYBINE is much nicer than the old one my dad had last time I tried to be a farmer. That was too long ago. Since the loss of my dad it never happened again. I never went back to the farm. Ever since then I never even went to a memorial service for a good reason, at least in my mind.

Thankfully the girls have bonded with the goldens and they are going to protect the girls while I am busy on the tractor. I can see they have been around dogs before and I'm more than sure Jack was a little spoiled before his terrible loss. They must have been heartbroken. The girls are in heaven today, and the goldens are in need of extra love so it's a win-win for everyone. In no time, I'm pulling into the first field and making my opening swath. It always seems strange to me going backwards for the opening round on the fields. As I made the first round, I started to listen to the CBC radio station. It's amazing how much information I can get listening to that informative station.

My day was amazing and I'm finally feeling at peace with myself. The world didn't need me to be the caretaker of others' lives today, or for days to come. I was driving a luxury tractor with very little stress but considerable responsibility. It's a different responsibility than saving lives. Today the task is driving around a 140-acre field making it just a little smaller with every clockwise round. After the first round, it's easy going as long as I am careful on the corners. I didn't want to make a mess of the field by leaving hay standing or bunching up the swaths. My job actually helps the person bailing the swath in about four to six days. As long as the weather is dry and there's a little wind, the hay will cure in no time.

Farming, despite its hardships and stressful days can also be therapeutic. The physical work, gave me time to reflect and work out some personal, emotional and spiritual debates. Once I got into the first couple of rounds I start to relax enough to let my emotional door open up and my mind started to clear. The sounds of silence or the constant sound of the tractor at the set RPM actually works to massage my body. Enough to let me reflect on the good and bad parts I have faced while dealing with others' pain and suffering.

The physical labour, the endurance required and the mental task are completely different from EMS to farming but the mindset has many similarities. Ironically for both professions we need to care deeply, have pride, be willing to multitask, and we need to give the little extras in many ways. I strive to be always performing a skill at the level of a perfectionist in order to make my world or the things in my grasp better than when I came along. I can't do either role half-heartedly and last very long. What helps me be a better person for one round of cutting helps me in the other profession in many ways I hadn't thought of before today.

The day slowly passes by and I feel that this is the mental and physical relief I have needed for a very long time. It's just too bad that my friend is having so much grief. I'm glad I could help him and his family out. I'm going to need to do this more often, I think to myself. I think I should plan to do this more as I would be helping my friend out and it gives me some much needed peace of mind as well.

The EMS work that I love and have a passion for is still as good as ever to me. But the system is slowly taking a toll on my life. Even if I still love the work, it's still hurting me. Over the last several years work is asking for more and more. The staffing or the new people coming into the profession are different from what they used to be with many staff working casual, part-time or with multiple services. The level of commitment to one service isn't the same as it used to be in my opinion. The respect for equipment, for the service and to the people is not the same in my eyes either. We see the population base has increased, the hospital overcrowding is worse, and the hallway medicine never happened in the past. The waiting to drop off our patients didn't exist years ago but now in the city, waiting in a hallway is a normal day.

We are seeing more and more tragic overdose calls with fentanyl, crystal meth and other designer evil drugs. Most, if not all, of the recreational drugs are very addicting, toxic and poisonous and are killing people before they get a chance to live life. The days we could just go to work and not be scared about being harmed or injured are long gone. Some days, the increased pay or the benefits don't compensate for the increased risk.

I wondered if the evil people or events are just seen as normal now. The level of respect for people in uniform isn't the same as it was in the past. Police, fire and all EMS are seeing the disrespect at all levels in our daily jobs. The overtime or the extra shift needed to help lessen the burden on our health care system is not therapeutic anymore. Despite my desire to help others and serve the public, there is always someone needing more and more out of us all. The more we give, the more people take from us and the less they try to help themselves it seems. Somewhere it has to stop or in the end we have nothing left.

After every round, I make another swath of hay that slowly makes my progress visible. But secretly as I complete another round and my task is slowly being completed I feel better about myself. As I complete my given task another layer of stress or anxiety comes off of my recent troubled past events. Many people will never know the pain of trying to save a dying baby, or the screams of a parent after their child has been killed or just died. Those sounds never go away, they lesson most times, but some calls never go away. Plus, responding to similar calls takes us back to the anxiety we felt. The pain of losing and the buildup of repeated suffering returns when we are not expecting it. I know that PTSD and compassion fatigue are definitely not understood very well within our profession. Every single person affected by the trauma they are part of has a unique way of unwinding or removing the stress and this important but physical task is my newest way to heal or provide self-help.

Today my HAYBINE just powers through the thick hay and the sections just seem to cut the field at exactly the right height. It's going well on my first day and even if I was lacking sleep, I feel rested and refreshed. About noon, my dinner arrives by Sally and her three little angels and right beside them are my amazing goldens. Sally has brought me an amazing home-cooked lunch. Then the dessert was to die for – it was sweet homemade fudge, the best I have ever had in my life. But something more special warms up my heart and it's the interaction of my golden retrievers with complete strangers. Before today they didn't know these little ladies but by lunch they have everything set up and everyone has a role or a job. In minutes after I arrived this morning the stage was set for love, safety and loyalty that does not happen in most situations. It is set up with no training or commands, just love. This type of situation rarely happens in life especially between people and animals. Tinsel is just one of the kids and Pebbles is the protector and watches everyone from a distance.

The love the girls all show me is without question and unconditional. My smile must be as big as my heart today. Seeing the girls playing with the puppies and them taking turns following each other around is so cute. Life could not be better for the girls right now, despite having their dad laid up resting on the couch. They are so loving and attracted to the affection from Pebbles and Tinsel. Funny thing is they keep getting special treatment from Tinsel and she shows no sign of getting tired of them. They keep getting Tinsel-hugs, which are her specialty. Tinsel just comes up and puts her head and shoulders on someone and holds it for as long as you let her. She shares love like no other dog I have ever met. We call it a Tinsel-hug. She's bonded with all of the little girls and stays with them all the time. Pebbles is very different and watches over the girls but always from a distance and from different spots to ensure they're always safe. Signs of a true faithful mother.

My lesson from this day is forming in my mind. The lesson of the day today is about feeling safe. When we feel safe we can open our heart and when our heart is open we lose our fear of the past. I can see it with the way Pebbles watches over the three girls. Tinsel plays with them and gets close and shows unreal affection but the more I drive around the field I can see an important lesson that maybe others take for granted. The girls can play and learn many things together as long as they are safe. With an open mind, we can seek additional adventures as well as learn at our own unique speed. Something to remember is that we all learn at different speeds and from different stimulation or interpretation of our sensory input.

I can see by how the girls interact and play they are quickly picking up new lessons, increasing their physical ability, learning how to play or create new pathways for friendships. It is so amazing but also funny how they just stick to Tinsel and absorb her energy, but with Pebbles they respect her and treat her like royalty. How do they learn that in just one day, I wondered? That is amazing as it just happened with no direction or planning. Pebbles set the stage, Tinsel follows the rules and the girls interact with each other just like team members with respect and caring attitudes.

But to be safe I think you need to feel wanted or perhaps feel worthy of being someone that matters. Pebbles, being the strong pure power golden retriever, knows how to give love. She also knows something else but it comes from within. I don't know how they develop it but when they are around good people they learn love, loyalty, 100% dedication to participate in all actions, and most of all they learn to forgive and forget transgressions so we start on a positive note at every interaction.

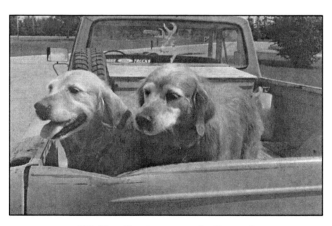

"Golden Retrievers to the Rescue"

Chapter 12: Recharging a Broken Spirit

"Saving Our Own Angels"

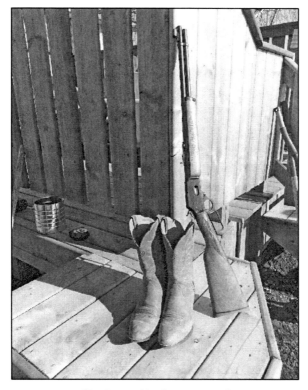

"Saving a Life that Matters."

We will sometimes need to look through the gates of hell for a true rescue mission. Someday someone we know there is in trouble but we can't always see it coming. Sometimes we won't see the danger until it's almost too late. No matter how good you are at being careful, some tragedies are just around the corner. Today I had been welding and fixing some broken farm equipment. The day had been so peaceful and I'd been completely immersed in fixing broken farm equipment since early morning. I had music playing in my head phones and no matter how hard my work was, I just kept working and I was pleased with myself, as I was making things work while the tunes just kept playing loud and proud through my headphones.

It's so amazing that with just the right equipment such as good torch, a six-inch side grinder, a drill press and a chop saw, that I could make anything I need as long as I have a little wisdom. Almost anything can be fixed when it comes to farm equipment as long as you have the metal parts and a good welder; it's the farmer's code. If you are a farmer you will need to be able to fix or repair almost anything because the garages will bring a person's bank account to nothing in a hurry. One trip to town to fix a tractor can easily be $8,000-$10,000. You can't *not* fix it, as you need it to make a living. I know Don has a great neighbour, Bill, who is a genius in electronics and with special hard repairs. He never charged a cent but in exchange uses the shop from time to time to fix his own equipment.

The grinding, the welding and the reinforcing of the metal is interesting. Some of my welding looks better than anything else I have done in my life. With the right welding rod, the right heat setting and the proper penetration you can make any two pieces of metal one for life. I think to myself this is wonderful. I just need some primer and some paint and it will be brand new. A few days of rain have slowed things down but the pastures need rain. I've had an amazing three weeks of being a farmer and rancher.

The goldens have had a better holiday than I have, I'm sure. Pebbles and Tinsel have made some lifelong friends as well as been spoiled rotten. The girls have spent every day with them while I put in long hours in the shop or field, fixing. Thankfully Don got a pool set up for the girls last week and nothing will keep Tinsel out for long – that dog is part fish. I have never seen kids laugh so much in my whole life. They have Tinsel diving to the bottom of the pool fetching rocks or toys.

Don is sitting on the deck, watching me help his family. He's told me he would not have been able to survive over the last several weeks without my help. He possibly would have lost it all in the end. "Thank God, we came to his rescue" he says, smiling from ear-to-ear. Every day I have found something extra to do around the farm. Looking back, I had not taken a day off but I had taken the kids for ice cream more than once, that's was for sure. Don told me that the last two years have really hurt them and now this. I told him it was nothing. I said the puppies needed a break from me anyway. He knows my dilemma and why I needed a holiday from working in EMS, seeing one too many bad things and understands that as well. So, in the end, we are helping each other heal. It's a win-win for everyone. I still think this was planned by someone higher than us all.

Don almost had forgot I was also a good welder and after coming to the shop and seeing my work, he gave me a raise. The reward was free beer in the shop fridge – even if I didn't drink much, it was there, cold and wet. Over the years while farming, I appreciated just one or two cold beers, and then it was back to work. But for the most part it was a non-alcoholic cold and wet drink. I had to be in the right mindset for a beer – never when I was sad or down. It was my golden rule. I didn't want to start or to go down that road.

On hot days, one or two beers would go down very smoothly and keeping the beers to a minimum kept me out of trouble with anyone. At least I wasn't an alcoholic, for if I was and in a high stress career I could see it becoming a tragic combination. It's not worth taking the chance for any reason. One impaired driving charge and I would lose everything. Many years ago, I went camping with my three kids, had one drink and everything was good. Heck, I had the kids get me one more and in an hour or two I wanted one more. My son looked at me sternly and said, "Dad, two is the limit." He was only about eight or ten years old but just like that, my night of drinking was over. Camping or driving was the same limit to them. I guess I made the rule and they had heard me say it more than once. I fell asleep without any chance of a hangover that night.

Don is on the mend and his doctor is proud of his progress. Sally had him set up on the outside deck in the shade keeping an eye on the farm and watching the livestock along the riverbanks. With the right medications, the right amount of rest, elevation of the infected leg and a compliant patient, healing is going ahead of schedule. Don was fortunate to have me as a friend. Don knew something of my personal struggles in fighting life and death so knew by him taking a break it was therapeutic for me. Don had said to Sally it was so easy to watch someone he trusted work for them, when he trusted his life and his family's life with me. That made it even more special after he told me about his feelings. It was the perfect therapy for us both and no matter how hard I looked at it I had come so much further ahead even if I missed two of my appointments for therapy which I had happily cancelled. The therapist had then talked to me twice in the evening by phone and also to Don at my request and with my blessing. I think she just wanted to make sure I was not hiding or running from hell but in no time, she understood and gave him the names of a few books for me to read.

The first one - *Overcoming Trauma and PTSD: A Workbook Integrating Skills from ACT, DBT, and CBT*. It was a paperback edition by Sheela Raja (2013). I reviewed it and was happy with the review. I asked Sally to order me six copies because it would be read from cover to cover and I needed a few for friends and for emergency situations as they arose. She reluctantly took my credit card only if I promised to come back for a free Christmas holiday with her family as a surprise to Don so we could have a better visit. The summary was: "The truth is that there is no right or wrong way to react to trauma" and we all have seen that in the past. Then it goes on to say: "There are ways that we can heal from our experience" or in my case I needed to "uncover my own capacity for resilience, personal growth and recovery." This had to come from me before I could go ahead in life. The overcoming of "trauma and PTSD offers proven-effective treatments." The book described our acceptance and commitment therapy (ACT), which scares me the most some days, then dialectical behaviour therapy (DBT) which I had no idea about so far, and then cognitive behavioural therapy (CBT) which I had read about in the past.

I liked the summary about the book that we need to overcome both the physical and emotional symptoms of trauma and post-traumatic stress disorder (PTSD). I'm sure we all have to deal with the physical and the emotional stress created caused by the mental concerns that the EMS life or the tragic events we were witnessing to help start healing. If we do not address the issues they too would fester, and over time it would take its toll on our life and also affecting our successful career. This book will help me address the stuff I can't share with others very well, or at all most days.

Sarah and I had talked about some of it but not all of it. I needed to find some relief from the painful flashbacks especially at night or during a call and the insomnia or palpitations I was experiencing before, during and after the calls. It includes worksheets, checklists, and physical or mental exercises to help me start feeling better and begin my journey on the road to recovery. I then thought about it and ordered three more. One for Sarah, Robin, and also for Ken because they could meet this problem head on early in their career and we would help change our culture. Then my final thought before I got back to work that day was that I needed to start to think of Christmas gifts for Don and Sally's angels.

In seconds, I had the idea. I texted Sarah and asked her to find me a pair of golden retriever puppies, preferably ones that are ready for a new home in a few weeks as that was when I was leaving. I asked her to make sure that we pay for them and then they can hold them until my last day of farming. The cost doesn't matter but have a look at them and ensure their disposition is 100% kid-friendly. I need a warrior and I need a gentle giant. I wanted to get females because they are so good with looking after people in my judgement. But in a pinch, I would take a male golden retriever as well, knowing I had one in the past and he was amazing. His name was BamBam; he was Pebbles' original partner as a protector and a real rural crime fighter.

Sarah acknowledged the text and said she was missing me but she had a good partner. She was booked with Greg who was one of the kindest, wisest but quietest paramedics within our service. He had backed us up on a few calls in the past and was a volunteer firefighter. Then I started to cry. Greg would have been the paramedic from the volunteer fire department who had helped to save my life. I didn't realize that until today. His wife was Becca, one of my best friends in ER and one of the best ER nurses in our hospital. The two of them made me smile just thinking that I had such good and loyal friends. I needed to thank him in a special way and I would find just the right way. My time on the farm had done much more than I dreamed possible. I had memories back that I had lost or blocked out for a very long time. They were scary but it was refreshing to bring them up and try to deal with them face to face. I had to dry my tears and go for a little walk around the farm before I was ready to go back to work. Today it would have to just wait for me. I know they would understand.

One night we had sat and had a beer in the shop after fixing the 2290 with a leaking hydraulic line and Don shared some of his personal problems. In the past, they had a few hired men over the years but not many were reliable. A few were outright dishonest and would not work on his farm ever again. The day I arrived they finally had someone they trusted and the kids got a new uncle who had taken them shopping and for ice cream a few too many times as well.

Chocolate dipped cones make friendships even stronger. The only tragic thing was Tinsel was sharing Aimee's cone and licked it until it disappeared in about three licks. The simple fix was to go and get one more cone and then everything was fine. I felt sorry for Tinsel as she gave me the saddest puppy dog eyes in the world. Well Tinsel knew better – even though she may have been offered a lick, she took it literally. I was a big sucker as I got both goldens one more ice cream cone. It was a hot day and looking back, they needed it.

The time on the farm was so therapeutic for me. When I was immersed in so many tasks that were meaningful it was slowly healing me from my past years of stress. It's almost like my soul was taken out, washed off all the badness and reinserted with a clean slate. The extra benefit was when I worked for a friend that appreciated anything I did and didn't second-guess my actions. I had no extra rules. A few times I had broken something or blown a hydraulic line and I never felt like I would get in trouble. We simply stopped and fixed it and carried on. All I had to do was just stop and fix it, and then go right back to work. I never thought anyone noticed except the neighbours driving past who stopped and came in for a little visit to make sure I was okay any time I was stopped or may have needed a helping hand.

One afternoon I pulled into a half section of hay and had made my first round when the tractor died. I had no idea what was wrong. I tried for about twenty minutes to find the problem and one of the local Hutterites came past and stopped to lend a hand. In no time, I had two more people come along and we were tearing the tractor down until we found the problem. It was a blocked fuel filter, which was common with bad fuel. I asked if they would mind giving me a ride to town to get a fuel filter and they were more than happy to help. On the way, the older gentleman who was probably the elder asked me some questions such as who I was, why I was visiting and then asked how Don was doing. I told him and he patiently sat there and quietly listened. He was a very quiet but thoughtful gentleman.

When we got to town I went inside and found a filter and I asked if I could charge it and they said sure. I thought about Don and Sally's last several years and then I thought about the stress of their last month. I thought again about charging it but it felt wrong. I knew they had a few unpaid bills and they were trying their best despite being knocked down. Before I left I had made a donation to a good cause and after I had left in a week they would get a "paid in full" notice. In some way, the Pebbles and Tinsel Consulting Service had looked after the bill. Harry just watched from a distance and never said anything but simply smiled and he knew my heart was pure and it was good. I knew that when they went to pay the bill, it would make them laugh about who paid the bill and then they would hold each other tightly. They would both cry and thank God for all the good people in the world. They would see the bill paid in full by Pebbles and Tinsels Consulting service.

Then Harry offered to take me for a quick coffee, which shocked me, as I was not a member of their colony and that honoured me. I politely smiled and looked at him and thanked him for his hospitality but especially for the ride and the extra help to fix the tractor. He just nodded and said it was nothing as we drank our coffee. Then I told him jokingly I had to get back to work or I would get fired. He laughed and said, "I don't think so." We were off and heading back to the field with our parts in hand. It was like we had known each other for years. In half an hour, I would be working again. On arrival at the field I was shocked. There were two identical self-propelled HAYBINES in the field and they were cutting up the field so much faster than I was used to seeing. I was shocked and humbled to know others were so caring and kind in this sometimes mixed-up, evil world. That was one of the kindest things I'd seen in a long time. They had their own work to do but when they realized someone else needed help they dropped what they were doing and they made Don and Sally's field their only priority. They had made themselves a new friend for life.

I would forever be grateful. Don and Sally would be buying chickens, jerky and garden produce from our new friends from today onward. That was how life was to be paid forward. When people needed help, others simply pitched in and made it right. In no time, we had the tractor running and I was cutting round and round with my new partners in farming. The elder just sat and watched us all from a distance and made sure we were doing okay. After a while he was magically gone from his parking spot. That was when I realized my tractor was full of diesel and they had surpassed any level of kindness I had ever seen between two neighbours. Then I smiled as even in his silence he had made small miracles happen while I was getting the fuel filter.

When you have good people around you they simply watch over the other good people around them as well. When something goes wrong they know as well that things are wrong and they intervene as needed. After all, they had been in the same spot in the past. One day I stopped and put the hood up on the tractor and in five minutes a passing farmer pulled up beside me. We both searched until we found the leaking hydraulic line and in no time, I was back in another stranger's truck and off to town. In two hours, the tractor was fixed and running again. I noticed it a few times when I was stopped in the middle of the field that if I didn't get going someone was checking on me. If it wasn't Sally, it was Don or it would be a random neighbour. I could not believe that we had places in the world that people really still mattered to each other like family.

They all cared for each other when people were in need. Everyone seems to notice everything and if someone needs help it just happens. For all the badness in the world, this one place in the universe is so relaxing and refreshing. It's powerful beyond anything I have ever seen being done in my life. This holiday had been an amazing adventure and it had cost me nothing more than fuel, treats for the kids, treats for the puppies and a few extra farm things that came out of Pebbles' and Tinsel's savings fund. I would just smile when

Don called me to give me grief about spending that much money on his shop equipment but it was my gift to the farm. It also made me more comfortable fixing my own stuff because I had helped purchase some extra needed tools.

Tonight, we were going to celebrate Don getting his last IV antibiotic treatment. In a week, he would be back to work and fortunately a few close neighbours will help him until he is okay to do things himself. My timing to come and help was perfect.

I was looking forward to tonight being extra special, as I made a phone call last week and after a little coaxing, my partner Sarah had packed up and come for a holiday on her extra week off. I promised her she would be looked after and I knew she would be spoiled rotten as well. Sarah also needed some time to clear her spirit. I knew Sally would treat her like royalty, plus I really needed to talk to her. Most of all I wanted to share my little part of heaven with someone that mattered to me more than life.

Sarah arrived yesterday around supper time. The girls had given her a royal tour with puppy supervision. They could not go anywhere without Pebbles being close by. Pebbles the Wolf and Tinsel the Terminator are the best in the world to look after the three angels in training. Tinsel made me laugh more and more as she was just playing and never seemed to get tired. If Tinsel wasn't getting wet or bugging kids, she was chewing on sticks. She never stopped chasing sticks and running in circles around everyone. Life is so precious it's worth sitting back and admiring it when you get the chance. Pebbles simply took the world in and stood her watch.

Sarah looked so different in her street clothes. At work or after work I have only seen her in her uniform. It's not that we couldn't get together after work; we just never made it happen. Now I can see her smile getting bigger and for a few hours the girls took turns going for rides. After watching Sarah with the girls, I realized she would make a great mom someday; she's so good with kids. Sarah was slowly looking around and seeing the world I referred to as heaven. The open spaces and the sound of silence were second to none. It was my new heaven. Even if it wasn't the real heaven it was much closer than I'd ever seen in my whole life. To watch the girls run and play and to see them smile so much while playing with Sarah gave me more hope for humanity. Maybe we had some hope yet for the future.

Today I had Sarah driving the big Case 2290 tractor for the first time in her life hauling big round bales. The tractor made the miles and hauled in load after load home from the field without a problem or a breakdown so it has been a great day. Sarah said she's never been on a farm before but she's a fast learner which I knew from the first time I met her. She was not like the normal urban lady that I knew from the city. Any task I asked of her she mastered faster than I could have, I was sure. She just radiated strength, confidence and had the determination that I had never seen in any partner in my whole life. I was lucky as I got the new 2011 Case IH Puma 145 CVT cleaning corrals and spreading manure with another 2390 Case tractor so it was not a bad day. It was not a pleasant job but as they say, manure happens. Regardless, I was getting it done and in a few more days one more chore would be checked off the list.

Thinking about it, there was not one task she could not master except maybe being mean or nasty to anyone. I never doubted her ability to master any task or skill from the first time I met her. Thankfully Don had a nice round bale hauler that works behind the tractor and in no time Sarah was bringing home fourteen heavy round bales every trip just like a professional. I watched her from a distance and it was the coolest farm implement I'd ever seen. It was amazing how it loaded and unloaded from the cab. Sarah never really had to stop or even slow down. With good solid tight bales, it made the task even easier. Sarah made me so proud to have asked her to come and share some of her valuable holidays helping out on this busy farm.

Looking at it as an outsider, Don and Sally had been granted a gift from both of us showing up and helping out. They were so happy as they knew they had gotten behind in so many things over the last few months. In no time, they were getting caught up and some extra work was also being done at the same time. With us both helping, things were getting done and the everyday jobs were also being done. One by one the tasks were being removed from the long list of summer chores they needed done. It was like one extended family helping everyone out with every job to make the farm more successful. Thankfully we had the time and the ability to give them both a much better summer.

Tonight, we are having a BBQ and then a bonfire so it will be a longer night than normal. Sarah is staying in the guest room with Sally and the girls spoiling her. So far, the goldens are with the kids until bedtime then with me till the next morning. Funny thing, in the morning they were lying by the truck waiting to go back for more love and spoiling before I was even dressed. They too are enjoying the working holiday.

While I was welding today, I had been thinking about Sarah and how she was just so special in many ways. I have never seen her swear or get down or upset about anything. I haven't seen her lose her cool at work even once. I wonder why she ended up in my life. It's not that I was not attracted to her because I was but not in a sexual or crazy seductive way. It's just like she was put on this earth as an angel, if that was possible and I wonder if it was just for me. Someday I'm going to ask her and she won't lie to me I just know. I was just not sure if I was able to handle the answer. Those considerations made me feel strange inside. My life sure has its moments of good times with good people all the way to the bad days to seeing the worst people imaginable.

Well maybe we can't prove angels exist or were real, but Sarah's my angel so it doesn't matter as the proof is in the person. It's so good to see my partner at my side constantly making me smile and helping me become whole again. Maybe tonight I can ask her and I will know the truth. I really want to find out more about her than I have learned up to now. I want to know where she was raised, her family life and how she ended up where she is today. I guess before today I was not ready, as I was scared to know too much. I think that was part of me not letting Lisa go or maybe scared to get too close to her in case something happened to her as well. I was not sure but I think there was something holding me back from asking. I just didn't know what it was so I never crossed that line.

I have never seen anyone like Sarah in the past. Lisa was so amazing but she was different from Sarah. I could not or would not compare them. They were both angels in my mind. I have not had time to visit with her yet but she gave me a special long hug after breakfast and said to me quietly "God I've missed you so much at work. I can't wait until we are back at work again." She kept looking at me and said, "we make one great EMS team." That meant a lot to me. It's something I needed to hear even if I hadn't thought about it. She then shocked me when she took one look at me and said, "The demons are gone, my friend." Then she turned and walked away. Then I knew without asking she was my guardian angel.

I suddenly realized she was right – they were gone. It took three weeks to turn my life around. I can sleep all night now which is something I have not done since my bad accident. I miss Lisa but not in a tragic loss type of feeling. It's like she's set me free with no regrets but I will always have a special place in my heart for her. Sarah had filled a huge void that no one but her could have filled.

I also haven't had any more bad dreams over the last several weeks. I've had no more times when I just wanted to give up on life after seeing repeated tragedy for so long. I can honestly say I was not suicidal but I also never really wanted to live. So, I guess that was one way to admit to myself I was in big trouble without feeling regrets or being embarrassed. I could admit that to Sarah and know she kept it all in confidence. I can and would trust Sarah with my life. Somehow my life had been given a second chance to get my life back together again. I could finally go back to work and know I had a chance to make my life normal again.

I can't believe how refreshed I felt inside. Over the last year, I had seen some serious ups and downs in life. Thankfully the right people came into my life and turned me around when I needed it the most. Ironically, my prayers did work even if I never told anyone, but someone must have been listening.

It seemed unfair or strange that Don had to get sick for me to get to this part in my life but that is how life unfolds some days. We can look for the good in life or we can keep digging up the bad things. Looking for good is easier and healthier. Thankfully Don is getting better and he's getting some good help on the side. His kids are being looked after by the killer goldens. Life is good. I think that things must happen for a reason.

I needed a mental health holiday and I bet my BP is much better. I'm sleeping so much better, so that's a good start for me. Almost all the reasons I needed help have been addressed over my holidays. The therapy I needed was received even if I had to relive some badness to bring out my negative feelings. All in all, it was one of the most effective therapies I could imagine possible for me and it didn't cost me much other than some fuel, some spending money and time to heal. Plus, my friends have a parts bill that is zero at a time when it means everything to them both. Thankfully they won't get that surprise until the end of the month and they can't blame me because I will be back in Alberta saving lives I hope.

Throughout the day, I have been re-living the good and bad events. By the end of the day I was in a much better place. My miracle was being put in this place of time, with just the right people. Slowly I can break down each bad call and pick it apart. In the end, it was destiny or divine intervention on many of the calls. Once someone is critically injured or they have been shot, the damage is done. We cannot or should not blame ourselves for not saving them because in the end it was out of our hands. Even with divine intervention or a trauma team at the scene we couldn't have saved them but we would have given them one hell of a run for the money invested, that's for sure.

The long days have definitely given me time to think. The next step in my healing was to sit down with Sarah and we were going to work on issues as a team, on things I was still having trouble with. I still had a few scary past events that even today I don't understand and can't wrap my mind around them at all. But tonight, is our night to relax so as I pull into the yard, my workday is done. Tonight, we are going to have a special celebration for Don. We can finally relax and enjoy the evening.

I parked the tractors after I had fuelled them all up so they would be ready for a new day at first light. The fluid levels were all good and the equipment was ready for a long hot day tomorrow. I had to shower and change to be respectable tonight and then I was ready to rumble. The goldens were more than happy to see me but Pebbles was not herself. She stayed a good distance from us while we had supper, which was not like her. She just stood away from us all, and watched us, she never seeming to want attention. I went over to her a few times to make sure she was okay. She looked okay but was just not herself. I thought I would watch her closely in case she was sick or had hurt herself. Time would tell and I would not hesitate to take her to the vet no matter what the cost. She was worth every cent. Somehow or by some strange reason Pebbles was guarding us all even if we never knew danger was close by.

The supper was amazing with some of the best hamburgers I have ever had. The kids made sure both golden retrievers had extra. Tinsel would not quit until I gave her the look, and then she stopped pestering everyone for repeat treats. I only could eat two, then I won't need to eat for two days. The puppies are also full of human food and after supper they were back sleeping beside me. Pebbles was still not right.

After some time, she came and stayed beside me, but she would not rest. The kids went out to play after supper while the parents and the big people were just sitting back and relaxing. It was very therapeutic for every one of us.

We were sharing stories and it was some of the most relaxing sharing I had seen in years between people. Everyone just felt so comfortable with each other. Over the next hour, the sunset and darkness was slowly advancing from the eastern sky. Tinsel was finally lying down at my side resting as she had run with the girls all day long and must have been tired. I looked around to see Don, Sally and Sarah in deep conversation about some of the life and death events from our past.

Tinsel was suddenly up and gone from my side. She was heading in a northern direction straight to the girls at a fast lope. Pebbles was now sitting up and she was looking to the southwest direction towards the river. Then Pebbles was off and running as hard as she could go towards that direction. She looked more determined than I'd ever seen her in my life. Thinking back, I would have been scared seeing her coming at me all forty-five kilograms of solid muscle. The kids were about 300 to 400 yards north west of the adults playing in a small group kicking a soccer ball around just having fun. I had not noticed much until right then but suddenly something was very wrong.

The goldens would not be moving so quickly for no reason – and in two different directions. It made no sense to me other than danger was close by. They have a mission. I always knew they were my guardian angels but no one else would ever believe me, except maybe Sarah. This is very serious; even if I can't see or hear danger, it must exist. Their sense of smell, hearing or special wisdom is why they are such good protectors. I looked at Sarah and she looked at me. I looked worried, she nodded but said nothing and she too started looking around.

Pebbles was picking up speed and was now running for her life. It was not like her to leave my side in the evening so something was really wrong. She was now running as hard as she could physically go. I had just been watching the kids play but suddenly I was worried. I didn't know why but it was something bad. I was slowly getting scared from the unknown I can feel but cannot see or hear coming.

I stood up and started looking back and forth in both directions as the golden retrievers ran. I can't see danger but the hair was standing up on the back of my neck. My heart started to beat faster and faster. My eyes were dilating and I was looking left, then right and back and forth. I had to tell myself to slow my breathing down. Today, lives were on the line. I can't see danger but it has to be close by. Trouble is pending even if I can't see it, must be just around the corner. Sarah looked at me and she too saw the fear in my eyes. We both figured it out at the same exact second and we told each other what to do without a single word. Sarah jumped to her feet and ran to my truck as fast as she could go. She knew what we both needed. Sarah had been out shooting with me a few times and she was an excellent shot which was what was needed in the next few seconds. It was time to save a life with lethal force.

At the same time, I ran in the other direction towards the deck of the house and grabbed my trusty old friend that was loaded and stuck up high in the rafters on a hanger after I came back from working. For a few extra seconds, I was trusting Pebbles and Tinsel with my friend's kids' lives and I must not or cannot be wrong.

I debated running to the girls but I didn't know what I was running into so it was a planned rescue. But it was with huge risk. I knew I needed my gun. This was the one reason I had a gun in my life - was to save a life – and it was happening tonight. I never shot anything for sport and I would not ever shoot anything for fun. One time in my life as a kid I aimed and shot something, I never forgot it. Even if it was something we could hunt, I had shot it for the wrong reasons. I would never do that again. That was not in my creed even if I had made a mistake as a kid. I had done something stupid. Everyone can learn from a mistake I know. I had and made sure I would be much more responsible from then on for a reason. After that day, all life had become more precious to me.

In less than ten seconds I had grabbed my 30/30 off the high shelf and was running full speed towards the hill straight to the girls. It was the highest part of the hill right by the valley that ran parallel to the river. Don had loaded it and put it up in case of need since my arrival after the predators killed Jack. Still, no one knew who or what the predators were but they existed. Sarah had already grabbed my .338 and was running towards Pebbles. Thankfully Sarah could shoot, as we had practised a few times. I realized the kick would most likely knock her backwards as I had specially loaded the shells for speed and to knock down bigger animals. That gun would stop anything that was alive on the planet. I just wished I had it, but I would settle for my old Winchester rifle any day as a backup gun.

I had to stop the pounding of my heart, which was calming down with my controlled breathing. I took another look towards the kids and I was lifting the gun at the same time knowing something was terribly wrong. Tinsel had reached Aimee and was pulling her backwards by the back of her dress as she started to cry out. She didn't understand why Tinsel was pulling her backwards. She was stumbling backwards and the other girls were yelling at Tinsel with their backs towards the predators most likely hiding in their now blind spot. Tinsel doesn't care about herself, she only cares for the girls. I had never seen such a heroic act in my life. Tinsel must have known she was in trouble too but it did not matter, as her life was optional if it meant saving her girls.

Pebbles was still running in the other direction for no apparent reason and was just cresting the river valley. Sarah was running after Pebbles at full speed. In a split second, I finally could see the massive cougar slowly crawling towards the kids. It's only about ten feet away from them. I aimed and shot at the same second. I had shot just as it was coming up to launch at the kids. There was no way I could have reached the kids to help them. I was only going to get one good shot. It was a hard shot as the cougar was in the deep grass but thankfully I had a little extra elevation on my side. In a split second my shot was free and I was chambering a second round. Time had seemed to be in super slow motion right now. I was scared, but strangely not afraid. I prayed I could not miss. This was a once in a lifetime shot. If I missed and hit a kid I too would die from the pain.

I had my precious Tinsel and three kids within a few yards of a predator that had already killed Jack. I could not let the cougar have even one chance at the girls as they would be killed instantly with the huge cutting teeth and powerful jaws. Tinsel would not have a chance against it in a one-to-one fight. Pebbles maybe, but it was just a maybe.

At the same exact second, I heard the death growl of Pebbles as she hit the second cougar with the force of a truck. Unknown to any of us as we had sat and visited, a second cougar was flanking the kids as a trained predator setting up a kill. This one was never in my field of vision. To this day, I will never know how the goldens knew trouble was coming. Even more, how they knew what to do to protect the girls without even a sound. I could not help Sarah just yet as it would be up to Pebbles the Wolf to intervene. I had to help Tinsel and make sure the girls were safe first and foremost.

My heart stopped when I heard my most valued friend's death growl. To me that was not a dog but a person tackling the cougar head on. It would be a battle for her very life. I knew in my heart she was big and strong but a cougar was a natural-born killer. Normally most people who get killed or attacked by a cougar never see it coming. It's a stealthy, fast and lethal killer. It has power, strength and stealth on its side. I didn't see it but Sarah had crested the peak beside the river and in a split second her shot was away as well. I would never have known it but Sarah was an avenging angel when she had no other alternative.

Everyone for miles would have heard the .338 magnum's deafening crack. I was praying Sarah's shot was true but in the back of my mind I knew Sarah was trying to hit a moving target that was fighting with Pebbles. It would be a fast-moving target. My golden retriever was in a battle for her life and so close she could also be harmed or killed by the bullet. The bullet was a massive heavy load but very fast-moving. It's was a special tipped 225-grain bullet traveling at around 3000 feet per second. It was a homemade special loaded bullet made for one purpose. It would reach out far, fast and kill anything in its path. My old friend Trabish had made the rounds for me years ago, for this one special reason. They were made to fly very fast and stay true for up to 1000 yards and today Sarah would show me they could pass the true test. Today one bullet could save one life by taking another. It was how life worked some days. It truly was good vs. evil today, I would have to say. Today we were not killing something for the wrong reasons; it was for the best reason in the world, it was for my best friend Pebbles the Wolf as well as Tinsel and three precious little girls.

As I was almost at the three girls, the first cougar started to rise. My shot had hit the animal but it was not a lethal hit and she was still alive. I stopped running and tried to aim for a centre mass shot. I was just pulling back on the trigger when Tinsel nailed her by the throat and flipped her over backwards. I started running towards them both and as soon as I could, I fired. Tinsel was not hurt and this side of the battle for three little ladies' lives was over. Thank God Tinsel had stood her ground. In the end, she saved Aimee and not my magic second bullet.

Now we had one down and one to go I was sure of it. At the same time as I fired my final shot, Sarah screamed out "Pebbles" and shot a second time. Don and Sally were running behind me and grabbed the girls for dear life. They were now finally safe. I was terrified at that exact second since I did not have time to help Pebbles. I was feeling so guilty as I turned and started running to where I had last seen them running over the crest of the hill. Tinsel got up uninjured and ran back to the girls and started licking them all. Aimee too had a guardian angel even if her Tinsel became a "Terminator Model" today. Who said there is anything wrong with an avenging angel, I wondered a few days later.

Now I had to turn my attention to Pebbles and Sarah. I was not sure what to expect but regardless I was going to find out right now. I could not and did not see any of the battle on Pebbles' side or what had happened when Sarah shot. When she had yelled and shot the second time, was the only time in my life I heard Sarah raise her voice. It truly got my attention and scared me even more to know it must have been for a reason. I had no choice but to trust Sarah to help Pebbles. The girls were all crying but unharmed and they were holding each other in a tight circle with Don and Sally over top. Tinsel was also now in the circle.

I turned and started to run towards Sarah and Pebbles. As soon as I crested the hill I could see Sarah was bending over Pebbles and I was too scared to speak. My heart must have stopped beating in my chest. As I got closer I could see Sarah was putting pressure on a big open laceration to Pebbles' front chest and to her left front leg. The massive cougar had two big holes in it and was dead. Pebbles looked my way and then put her head back down. She had done her job and then some. Sarah looked at my worried face and said quickly "She will be okay. Pebbles got him. I just finished him off." I then noticed the cougar was torn open at the front as well. It must have been a vicious battle but my lady won. Sarah asked if Tinsel and the girls were okay and I said they are all okay. I didn't have time to tell her our scary story just yet. That would wait for another time. Pebbles was the only thing in the world to worry about now.

Sarah was holding pressure and petting Pebbles gently and telling her, "You're okay, my lady. Today you earned your name Pebbles the Wolf." Tinsel was maybe a lot smaller and not as strong but tonight she was also one of the true saviours. I suddenly realized I was crying and holding Pebbles and now Sarah had two patients. Sarah looked into my eyes and her look told me without saying a single word. I said, "Thank you" without even a sound coming out for I could not even talk. Thank God, the girls and Pebbles were okay. It was one of the most courageous battles by the two most loyal friends I'd ever had. Tonight, I learned a new type of fear and hopelessness. But in the end, my faith in my friends proved to be as solid as anything I'd ever seen. Tonight, my faith in the good of people showed me others such as Sarah, Don and Sally mattered.

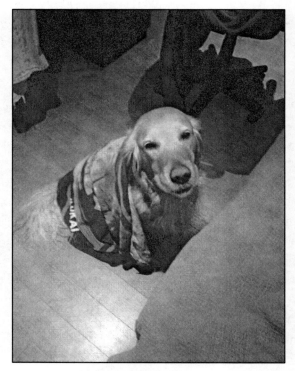

"Tinsel the Terminator to the Rescue"

"Putting Us Together Again"

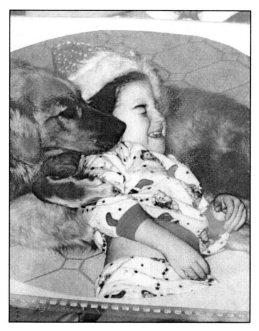

"Protecting the Ones, We Love"

Sometimes the benefits of us getting hit and our pathways in life being challenged is to keep others safe. Tonight Pebbles, Tinsel, Sarah and myself had done everything possible to save the lives of the little people that mattered. It was now our turn to help save Pebbles' life. In no time, the girls were quickly taken to the house with Tinsel making sure they were all safe. Sally and Tinsel stayed with the girls. They were still very upset but they too knew Pebbles must be hurt and keep saying and crying, "Mummy, Pebbles hurt." Sally told them, all "She will be okay." She then told them in a mummy's loving voice, "Pebbles has the best paramedics in the world helping her tonight. Tonight, Tinsel will keep us safe, my girls."

Don quickly drove the truck to the site of the final battle to rescue Pebbles. He found some towels and a blanket to help stop the bleeding and we used a blanket to carry Pebbles to the truck. Pebbles really now needs a veterinarian and Sally is on the phone right away, calling a family friend. In no time "Janelle" who is the local vet was notified. Janelle thankfully works in a mixed practice of big and small animals and can fix anything. Pebbles is rapidly carried into the back seat of the truck with Sarah holding direct pressure. The bleeding has slowed down and is not getting worse. Don ran back and grabbed the rifles. Sarah never let off from holding the dressing tight on Pebbles. At the same time, she's keeping her eyes on me to make sure I'm okay too. In no time, we're speeding away. Don is driving and I was on the other side holding Pebbles. The predators will be dealt with later so the girls will never see them. Janelle might want to see them and we will involve the local game warden to dispose of them, I was almost positive.

I always knew Pebbles was a fighter and this night proves it. Janelle will meet us all at the clinic with her assistant. In no time, we are speeding down the gravel road heading towards town. No one says anything for the whole trip. As we roll up to the local veterinarian clinic the door opens and our friend is waiting and ready for our injured warrior. Pebbles was taken right in and put in the treatment room. Janelle immediately took charge and in no time Pebbles was under her expert care. In the whole episode, there was not one growl or threat to anyone even if she must have been in severe pain and we were hurting her by moving her to get help. With the help of her assistant at her side they made Pebbles chemically sedated and more comfortable. In no time, they were examining the wounds and stopping the bleeding. Janelle slowly washed, cleaned and repaired the damaged tissue. It was time-consuming suturing the nasty lacerations. Pebbles was in the best place in the world to be saved. I could relax and know she would be okay.

Pebbles was given IV fluids; additional sedatives, as well as longer-acting pain medications and IV antibiotics were initiated. Over the next hour, the nasty mess was repaired. When it was all done, Janelle told us Pebbles needs to stay for few days to be sure she was going to be safe from early infection or shock. Pebbles was safe to rest and I'm sure she knew Tinsel would look after the girls in her absence.

Tonight, Pebbles was the hero and heroes are treated like royalty. She needed someone who could ward off any complications. Don insisted on paying all the expenses but Janelle won't take a cent. Janelle has heard the story of Tinsel and Pebbles tonight and they will never need an appointment at her clinic ever again. They have earned special treatment privileges and royalty care for life. Without their supreme protection one or all the girls could have been injured, or worse, killed tonight. Tonight, evil was defeated with blood, sweat, and pure love.

Pebbles was sleeping in a special room for recovery. Everyone was sent out so she could get some much-needed rest. I went over and thanked Pebbles for saving the girls tonight and as I turned to leave, I noticed Don in the doorway crying and holding Sarah's hand. Sarah also had tears coming down her cheeks which I walked over and wiped off with my hand and bent over and hugged her. I quietly whispered in her ear, "You're one hell of a shot my friend," and I held her tight. I could feel her heart beating against mine. Tonight, our heartbeats were as one. We were one-for-one on saving each other in times of need. Two hearts and the love that is created is what we need to make this world a better and safer place tonight.

This was one remarkable lady. Only I would ever know how special she really was because she would never acknowledge her achievement, as that was not Sarah at all. Tonight, she had saved my best friend from a vicious cougar attack that was almost twice as big as Pebbles. If it wasn't for her perfect shot our night would be a terrible heartbreaking one. Thank God for miracles. Tonight, there was more than one miracle in the air. The whole evening turned out as well as it could have, despite Pebbles' injuries. They would slowly heal and we would be at her side to take her through the bad days in the next few weeks. Sarah, Tinsel and Pebbles were the real heroes. I was just the backup plan.

I thought about the events that have transpired over the last several weeks and then I thought about the real angel, Sarah. Sarah had never let me down. No matter what the world throws at her, she adapts and makes the best out of the bad times. During the good times, she simply smiles and glows like no one I have ever seen in my life. During our bad days, she's strong, determined and solid as a rock. She has more character and endurance than anyone I'd ever met.

Our paths were meant to cross even if only a few knew our personal history. I could not figure it out but somehow there was a purpose in our meeting. She was my miracle and I was hers. Our paths were meant to cross at just the right times and it was nothing you could explain to anyone who had no faith in people and in humanity. Not only has she helped save my life, she most likely saved Pebbles from a terrible fate as well.

I looked at Don who was even bigger and stronger than I would ever be and he was also meant to be on our path of life's adventures. I gave Don a huge hug and I told him, "I think it's time to find you a pair of golden retriever puppies, my friend." I turned and thanked Janelle once more and we were off to retrieve and dispose of the predators. Our night was going to be okay as we had just the right people in our world that needed to be on our side. We were an unstoppable team.

In a few hours, we have the task done. The cougars were heavier than I expected. The male was almost 80-kg and the female was heavy at close to 50-kg, which is heavier than any golden retriever. Pebbles was 45-kg and Tinsel was 27-kg which is a runt but she was all heart and full of love for anyone but a predator. Thank God, the goldens triggered their safety mechanism and thankfully the rifles were close enough to prevent the events from being a real disaster. We had no extra seconds to spare and every second was used wisely tonight. Most people measure close encounters in minute or hours but tonight it was one-tenth of a second that mattered as well as a few perfectly placed lifesaving shots.

Normally the guns are locked up but since the loss of Jack I had been expecting the predators to come back. I thought it was most likely a pack of wild dogs or perhaps coyotes – I never even considered cougars. That's when I found out I was wrong. They are rare but still live across every province and territory across Canada. They will attack pets, kids and full-grown adults. I would never have expected them in this area, as they were normally about sixty miles further away according to an old trapper I had met in the area. Tonight, we made history for more than one reason, as it would be a night not forgotten by anyone involved for a lifetime.

On arrival at the farm, Sally made Sarah and I feel very welcome with a special hug. She had a few tears but never said anything but a very quiet and sincere - thank you - as we exchanged with her our caring smiles. She took us to see Tinsel and the girls. Tinsel was snuggled in bed with all three girls. It was so moving to see every girl had a hand on Tinsel even though they were all asleep. I went over and thanked Tinsel with a hug and she came to the edge of the bed and gave me a special Tinsel-hug. Then she went right back to lie with the girls while watching my every move from the corner of her eye. Tonight, I would be more than happy to sleep with my dreams or nightmares. I would say a special prayer for everyone especially Pebbles before my day was over. I just hoped that the girls wouldn't ever be scared of Tinsel or other dogs again. We told Sally that we would see them in the morning and Sarah offered to drive me to the trailer. Then she would come and sleep in the spare room beside the girls as added protection.

Sarah parked in the spare farmyard and then walked with me to the side of the trailer just after midnight to make sure I was going to be okay. We just sat and watched the stars for an hour and enjoyed the quiet times and each other's company. Thankfully, Pebbles was in good hands so I could stop worrying about her right now and Tinsel was not going to need backup tonight. I knew that Janelle would make sure Pebbles is safe tonight. Slowly I broke down and told her how scared I was when I heard her yell and then heard the second shot that terrified me even more. Her shots were both true, she had made a one in a million shot count for both shots. I was so thankful I too had held it together long enough to shoot true and steady. We both shared our appreciation of each other. I was so glad we each had what it takes in times of trouble to protect our most valuable possessions. The valuable possessions tonight were the lives of the kids and the goldens who were equally important to everyone involved. People who have never felt the love of an animal have missed out on one of the most valuable parts of living. Pure love with no reservations was the only phrase I could think of to describe it.

Sarah turned to me, as she was almost ready to leave and held me tight. I could see tears in her eyes. This lady is the only person in my whole life that seemed to understand my real feelings. This was the only person who could hear the messages from the special music that I play over and over. It was the music that reached into my broken and messed up heart to give me some peace and healing. No other person had ever taken the time to listen to my playlist on YouTube that I had ever seen or known. Sarah could feel the music therapy as well. Maybe it was meant for both of us to hear. Every person on the planet needs one true loyal and trusted friend.

I was so happy to have someone as a true friend for life, with no attraction other than pure love for a special friendship and no desire to have physical contact. Sure, I thought she was attractive, but she was more like an angel who was about the same age as my own daughter. In many ways, she was like my own daughter's best friend so I would do anything to keep her safe. The strangest feeling was that she was doing the same thing for me. I felt she was my guardian angel and she treated me like I was her superman. I just didn't know why so I simply asked her and I knew she would never lie to me. I just had to know the answer. There had to be something special but for the life of me I could not figure it out. Tonight, I was about to learn a lifetime of secrets that had never been told.

Sarah then told me her story. She was about six months old when I picked her and her mom up at a local motel in town about twenty-five years ago. She said she got the records after she turned eighteen because she was an adopted child by then and like many others she needed to know or try to find her mom if possible. She needed or wanted to know the story. According to the court records, EMS was called for a sick baby. On arrival, I could find nothing wrong with her but her mom was intoxicated and she was acting a little strange that day. We could have cancelled but I said let's go and we loaded them up and we were off. My partner would have just said okay and we were off to the ER in no hurry or no real reason to expect any complications at all as nothing was obviously wrong other than a strange feeling.

So, looking back with "me being me" we took her to the local ER for no reason other than I didn't feel good about leaving her. Even though apparently, I had no other reason. After I had given report and put them both in an OPD room I went to clean up the unit and finish my PCR. All of a sudden something was wrong. I could not see anything or hear anything but I knew something was terribly wrong. Something must have forced me to go back to that room but for some strange reason I just dropped what I was doing and went right back to the OPD room. I just had to go. I went back to the OPD room for one last look but I was not sure why but I had to go. The picture I saw I will never ever forget in a million years. I had a slight second of confusion and then fear at the same time and then I became superman. I was looking at a child being killed and it was happening right in the ER. I would not let this little girl be killed. Not on my watch. I would not hesitate to do anything possible to save the life of a child.

I yelled out as loud as I could and ran right at the mother. I was looking at a mother strangling the little angel right in the ER. As I got to her, a nurse came around the corner running and I grabbed the arm that was around the little girl's neck and pulled it away. I somehow did not care if I broke the arm or if it came off but I was freeing the girl at lightning speed. As I pulled the arm hard it released the little girl's neck and she fell into the nurse's waiting arms. We were both in the right place in time to save a life that day.

Little Sarah looked lifeless but she was free. I took the mother down rather forcefully and held her down. Multiple other staff came running and the little girl was immediately taken to the trauma room and resuscitated. Little Sarah was saved from death by the right interventions. The RCMP was present in minutes for backup as well as the on-call social worker that came running to help out. The mother was arrested and just like that Sarah had no more mother. She was placed for adoption and that was the end of the story but it was not the end of the whole story – it was just the beginning.

Sarah looked at me and said, "All my life I knew I was lucky and blessed to be alive. My adoptive parents were made aware of my near-death experience and they made extra effort to show me more love and attention than most children. They raised me as an adult in a child's body. When I became old enough to go to secondary school I always knew I would be just like you even though I didn't remember you or know you at all. I felt your presence beside me my whole life. After I got my first job as an EMR I found out who you were and tried to come here for my practicum. The first day I met you as your student I knew I had known you my whole life. You are my real-life superhero. After being your student on your unit I knew I could see by how you treated Lisa you were special. I knew someday, someway, I wanted to work with you. You always treated people right. Lisa and you were one of the most caring and dedicated people in the world in my eyes." I also felt the great loss after the accident for I too had special feeling for Lisa. I knew that accident would have hurt you but when you awoke and Lisa was gone it would break your heart in half. Somehow you made it through that most painful event.

Looking back Sarah had just given me faith that what I had done in the past was for all the right reasons. As long as I was alive and as long as I live, Sarah was now going to be that much more special to me. Now that we worked together and I was partnered with Sarah, I would have someone I could always know and trust to be at my side. I would do anything to keep her safe and out of harm's way at any cost for as long as we lived. As we sat and shared our special friendship I finally found peace in my heart for the crazy past I have fought for years. I had finally understood why I worked so hard to help people. Why I was so dedicated was that somehow, they all mattered more to me than my own life.

Tonight, was meant to happen, just as so long ago our paths had crossed and with the right interventions, life was spared. We had a destiny to fulfill at each other's mercy in the right moments of time. Tonight, I would sleep and the normal nightmares wouldn't have a chance to surface. Tonight, the evil was destroyed and we won a major battle. It was time to call it a day. I made sure Sarah got home, was inside my friend's house and the lights went off before I drove back to the camper. Regardless of the excitement over the last six to eight hours, I was soon dreaming and it was not the nightmares – it was about living again.

Over the next few days everything slowly went back to normal. Tinsel met me in the doorway to the kid's room in the morning and she made sure I had a good day when she was not looking after the girls. A few days after, Pebbles was able to come back from the vet and lay resting on the porch steps watching us, but resting and slowly healing her injured side. When she was well enough to travel, we would get her home. Sarah would help me get the pair of precious goldens safely home. In another week, we would be back on shift together saving lives.

As I was falling asleep, I made sure to remember in the morning to call the golden retriever breeder where I got Pebbles and check on the two puppies we needed as soon as possible. I had just found a home that needed some special people in their lives. They would have to be special to look after the three little angels and I knew they would have the right temperament and a superb attitude. Sarah and I would make the right arrangements over the next several days to get them to the farm. We had already ordered the puppies and we would make sure they were picked up and ' delivered. We would come back a few times a year to spoil them rotten. They would be raised to protect the girls – they too would be two very special living angels.

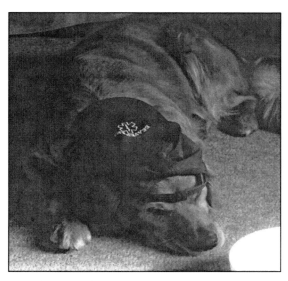

"Pebbles the Wolf – The Avenging Angel"

Chapter 14: Knowing When to Let Go

"Sometimes We Lose"

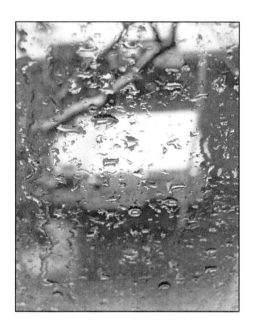

Admitting that we are losing a battle for a life as we struggle to reverse the causes and just stop treatment, to lose are two very different things. There are certain calls that are doomed right from the start. Regardless, we go and sometimes are forced or pushed to go on even when hope or logic is not on our side. The biggest example of this is a pediatric code. Sometimes we want to help and we need to help.

Sometimes the end is the right outcome in certain circumstances, even if we can't or don't want to admit or see it. On other calls, we end up quitting for other reasons a lot easier, such as mortal injuries our patient's bodies are inflicted with or the elderly for obvious reasons. They have had a good long life and we have no hope of saving them. It's much easier stopping CPR on an eighty-seven-year-old than a six-year-old, I can say without any regrets. We still feel upset but it's not the same in certain cases. Some cases hurt more than others and when they come along you don't forget them for years to come or you may never truly be able to forget them.

All in all, if you have survived your time in EMS you will have done your fair share of calls to see the good and the bad outcomes throughout time. Every once in awhile, we are challenged to reach our optimal functioning capabilities and we perform heroic skills. Then lives that should not have been saved will be spared and but some will not make it even with what seems to be such trivial injuries. We can't predict every outcome but we try to predict when a bad outcome is expected. Mostly, what we call preventable deaths are the harder ones to face alone. That is why we work as a team, we respond as a team, we do our best and in the end, we come home as a team. With the right team, regardless of the outcome we do our best. We demonstrate empathy and try to show compassion to every patient. Even towards the ones that really don't deserve it, or are not entitled to respect. There are some people closer to being evil than ever good at certain times in life.

Many people have a set rule on who attends or who drives. I think we need to be more flexible and more accountable for the outcomes. On some calls, I attend due to the nature of the call. On other calls, Sarah attends and we try our best to let the right person be in charge of the right patient. Sarah is an angel in disguise for some special calls, therefore she gets to attend. When we have rough and nasty people, I attend whenever possible. We all have our special attributes. I was always big and tough, where Sarah was and is always calm and seemed so much smaller and less intimidating.

I never really thought about our unique traits until we were driving back from the farm. On the way home from the farm, Sarah brought Pebbles so she could lie out better and relax with her soft soothing nature. I on the other hand brought Tinsel in the front with me in order to have an extra spotter for trouble. It was Tinsel looking out for Pebbles and Sarah watching me for the long drive home. Sarah ensured that we were all safely back home with Pebbles and all set up with the comforts of a five-star hotel before she went home herself. Pebbles needed a few more days to rest, as she wasn't healed up yet, she was still on vacation in my mind. Tinsel, on the other hand, patrolled the house and kept busy herding me around as I tried to clean, do laundry, unpack and get everything back to normal as soon as possible. It was then I found the three girls had made pictures of my golden retrievers and put them in my suitcase. That made me smile and hug my puppies one more time. I was trying to get ready for my first shifts back and looked after Pebbles, but she mostly stayed on the couch, which was her favourite spot in the daytime, and on my bed at night. Tinsel had then been promoted to the door guard for the night shifts.

Sarah was helping me with taking Tinsel for runs several times a day. We had Chris from the hospital and her two kids set up to take turns looking after them both when I started back to work. They would not be left alone until Pebbles was back to normal even though Tinsel was a pretty good guard dog on her own. Pebbles just needed extra care and love. I was so happy when I got a picture of the girls with two new golden retriever puppies. Thankfully Don and Sally had received the pair of goldens that will now be part of their family for years to come. They now have "Lily and Daisy" as the welcoming party for any bad guys who come along. The girls got the privilege of naming them. It was easy to see they loved flowers. Life will work out for their family with Don back at work, Sally is busy with the little ladies and now the puppies. They texted that they missed us both but were very thankful for our time and interventions. It was all meant to happen and it sure worked out better than it could have, all things considered.

On our first day back, Sarah and I were happy to be back to work after our time off. Sarah was more than happy to keep me out of trouble. I had been cleared to work as long as I could keep sleeping and handle the calls, so it was golden. I was not scared of much but some calls were always going to be my nemesis. The pediatric bad trauma or the pediatric codes, the dead kids and any neonatal codes were my worst. Everything else was just a normal day in hell I would have to say. Thinking back to the other codes I could not forget were the hangings. They were such a waste of life; many were so young. They had not even begun to live yet. I just needed a few easy weeks to help get my game face back and everything would be fine, but that wasn't going to happen. I should have known better. Karma had it in for me. I was going to give it a 110% fight no matter the reason. It was not fair to Sarah because she had to work on the harder calls and keep me out of trouble at the same time. That was unfair but we were a team despite our handicaps and limitations. I could not share with her all my good and bad days. It was refreshing to know I was not being put on trial or ever being judged. It came to be expected we would talk about our bad calls when the time was right. We were a winning team. She was my soulmate for EMS and I was hers for life from start to finish.

Right after lunch 9-1-1 called us because an Automatic Fall Detection system has triggered our dispatch. Sarah was driving and I was trying to figure out the best route, backup and what to expect on the way to the call. The call came in as a patient with an advanced type of Alarm Force system had apparently fallen. The dispatcher could hear someone in distress in the background with acute SOB over the Alarmforce system but with no speech or audible sound. Thinking about it, we could have a broken hip, an acute stroke or cerebral vascular emergency, a bad laceration or a severe breathing emergency so I was thinking about the worst possible problems, expecting and praying for the least on our arrival. We would not know until we arrived. I hoped it would be just a simple lift-assist but that was not to be today. Today karma came to visit us and brought its evil friends.

En route, we are notified our second unit is busy and if we need back-up it's twenty-five to thirty minutes away. The closest EMS service was being sent but we could use a Fire Medical Response with a much quicker response which I said was a better idea and they toned them out immediately. All we knew was we had a forty-three-year-old female with severe SOB at her residence. On arrival, we parked as close as possible and made sure we had access with the stretcher to enter the walkway. We grabbed our kits along with our monitor, placed them on the stretcher and made our way to the front door. In the distance, we could hear the co-responders who were in the fire rescue trucks coming in the distance. They had a high-pitched siren that was very distinctive compared with all other EMS vehicles. It always made my heart speed up for a second and got my immediate attention.

We are so thankful today that our backup was already dispatched and coming to help even before we arrived on scene. All we had to do was figure out what we were walking into first. Second, we had to quickly decide what our best treatment plan was on scene. Third, we had to decide what could we do en route on our short list of things to get done ASAP. What we found on scene still makes me shake my head in sadness and always will. Even if it's expected, death can always leave a mark on our soul.

We never expected such a mess when we opened the front door. We found our patient collapsed on the ground about five feet from her oxygen tubing. She was as blue as blue could be and she was barely breathing. It was mostly ineffective gasping for some lifesaving air of any sort. It looked as though she had fallen and her life alarm had automatically dispatched EMS. But where she fell her oxygen did not reach because it was down two stairs into the living room. She did not have the strength or the ability to get back up the stairs after the fall.

We looked at each other and sprang into action. I grabbed the BVM and Sarah grabbed the oxygen tank. In seconds, we were ventilating her with oxygen and assisting her ineffective breathing. Her colour was terrible and her heart rate was rapid and ineffective around 170 bpm. This lady was in serious trouble. She was what we would call a pre-code event. She was in severe respiratory failure leading to a pending cardiac arrest and it was happening right now.

I tried asking her about her goals of care as I suspected a bad illness as because she was on home oxygen but we had nothing to go on. There was no family and no medical alert bracelet. So, my only plan was to do everything. She was too sick not to help and if she had an advance directive I would have gladly followed it. Today we had no choice but to respond and attack the obvious life threats. I let Sarah ventilate while I applied the high flow nasal prongs. I knew this would deplete our oxygen in minutes. The fire crew walked in and immediately started helping. One of them was applying the monitor. Another was setting up an IV, as another one of them started the IV, as he was an EMT. Even if he had not worked for our service he was still registered and trained. Today we were but one team with only one patient as our only priority.

As soon as fire had arrived I told them we need to move to the unit as quickly as convenient but we needed an airway, then we needed effective breathing. A lifeline IV would be amazing and I wanted to see the monitor results for the Sp02, C02, BP and heart rate, which was very fast. One of the members went out and got a spare oxygen tank just in case. I knew we were using about double the oxygen we normally used so we had only half the time before our tank would be dry.

She would take an OPA right now so I elected to intubate her with nothing. Her ETCO2 was 86, which are crazy high, and her oxygen saturation was less than 50 when we started, slowly rising after we started ventilating. We had the suction set up and in seconds I was passing the tube. As I got her intubated I noticed the Sp02 was over 88 and the ETCO2 was less than fifty so we were heading in the right direction. Once we could ventilate her effectively we could decrease the oxygen use as well. The cardiac monitor was on and it showed a sinus tach but it was still too fast. Then the next problem hit us. The BP was 52/32 which is terrible. I thought we needed fluid, followed by Levophed® which most EMS will simply know as norepinephrine as the heart rate is too fast for dopamine at this time. But before any chemical pressor agents we needed to think of IV fluid so back to fluid I went in debate mode in my head.

I thought she looked dry and the best idea I had for that was IV boluses. As I listened to her chest I noticed almost no sounds at all in the right chest but not bad in the left. I wondered about that and I percussed her chest which was dull to percussion. That told me it was most likely fluid and not air. Now I was pretty positive we were in big trouble with her and we needed to get going.

By the look of her presentation I would bet she was an advanced lung cancer patient but I had nothing to prove it and we couldn't find her medical history. If we searched her bathroom or other spots we might find something. We found her purse with identification but that was it. As soon as we arrived at the local ER they would be able to pull up her history. Sarah was okay ventilating so I left her at that. She said it was difficult but manageable at this time. I passed her some Ventolin and told her to try it as right now we have nothing to lose and everything to gain. She applied it down the BVM through the special port and sure enough in a few minutes the oxygen levels were climbing and the breathing was easier with the BVM. Next, we had to get the heart rate down. Her temperature was 35.9 – hypothermia – which could be a little exposure, thyroid problems but most likely a severe or a septic (systemic) infection. The blood sugar was also low at 3.1 which isn't too bad but still low. Sarah was pushing in the IV fluid and added half an ampule of D50W and we can recheck the BGL in a bit. I started to think of a pressor for the low BP but had to let the fluid try to correct the heart rate and the BP as well. It all took time and we needed to move to our unit ASAP.

It was time to transport. We took a scoop from the unit; we all gently picked her up and placed her on the stretcher. I had already asked the fire captain for a driver and they were glad to help. Normally if this was someone without a terminal disease I would have called for STARS but today we had to wait and let the ER physician decide on the most appropriate care. We just didn't know so either way we were doing our best. I was positive we were doing the best for our patient under the current circumstances. If she had an advanced directive we would have crossed that line most likely after we arrived and intubated her. It is never a perfect world for us. Many days we arrive in grey or not so clear situations and we make the best of it. Rural EMS needs to problem solve and make decisions, as we don't have the luxury of backup just around the corner.

Thankfully we would have a short transport time and being a small hospital, they would find a solution for our patient in minutes. Many times, the ER doctors are family physicians and they often know the patients. Working rural EMS has its benefits as well. The best part of rural EMS in my view is the cooperation from the local police, which in many cases for us are the RCMP who many know us well, and the volunteer firefighters are very helpful to the EMS crews. It was an ideal team of people who magically got along and did the job as good as any urban professional teams.

Then the really helpful aspects of patient care are the local ER nurses and hospital staff. They do anything and everything to accommodate us 24/7. We very rarely wait for a bed in ER. They find us one. In the city, I've seen triage nurses put us at the back of the line because we were not an urban crew. That made me really sad for our rural patients with no ambulance for sixty miles but that was the way it worked. One day many years ago, I voiced my concern to an urban supervisor and I was told very directly and clearly that Urban matters, Rural does not. That didn't sit well with me. I thought health care should be uniform and equal but it is not and never will be in the system we currently live in today.

After we left scene I initiated a Levophed® infusion and was titrating it up as fast as possible with the BP dropping still. I was almost thinking maybe we should start CPR when we pulled into the local ER. We patched as an unstable patient saying we needed help on arrival. That was enough for the nurses and doctors to get ready. On arrival, the ER doctor met us coming in, asked a few questions and quickly turned and pulled up the Netcare records. We were hoping for some good news but sadly we all knew without any discussion it was looking very bad. Sometimes we lose before we start and today was a prime example of a bad situation with no good outcome in sight.

We transferred care and the nurses expertly took over and inserted a second IV, a Foley catheter and an oral gastric tube. In three to four minutes the doctor was back and closed the door behind him. Then he broke the very bad news to us all: stage four lung cancer, which is most likely from metastatic breast cancer. She was waiting for her Cross Cancer assessment and initial treatment. According to her radiology report she is full of cancer and there is no advanced directive. He called for a stat CXR and the initial lab work was done. The family have been notified. I have a call into her family physician. We should get a call back right away. Sadly, everything we just did was in vain and the outcome was meant to be terrible right from the very start of the call. When she fell she was already in distress which was most likely the reasons she fell in the first place.

While waiting, I started searching the statistics and I was shocked to see in 2012 some 16,000 cases were reported of cancer with over 5,000 deaths just in Alberta. I had no idea that breast cancer was a leading cause of death in women twenty-five to seventy years old with an increased incidence in older women. Out of that number, breast, prostate, lung and colorectal were the leading causes. That is the population of a small city. I never knew it was so bad. I was trying to write my ePCR and wondered how someone could get so sick and still not be receiving active treatment. Then I realized denial, poor health care for certain population groups, incompetent practitioners and the biggest problem – increased waiting times for diagnostic care and surgical intervention – all are poor due to our inefficient healthcare system. What made me extra upset is knowing WCB can get almost immediate care and they get priority spots in radiology procedures and then our country can say we don't have a two-tiered healthcare system. I beg to differ on that myth.

Shortly the family physician called the ER doctor back and a plan was made. After the family arrived and the situation was explained, care would be withdrawn. The patient had already requested to be treated as a palliative patient and the paperwork was not yet finalized. Regardless of her age, we had done our best in a terrible situation. Afterwards we asked to speak to the ER physician and went to find a quiet spot. Sarah and I sat down with him and I apologized for what we had done.

He said, "Stop, that was no one's fault. It was just bad luck all around. I feel bad for you both as you responded and walked into a big mess. I would have most likely done the same only I would have called STARS without considering the situation. You get to see something we take for granted. I see them presented and packaged in ER which is remarkably much different." Sometimes we all get to face a losing battle but we all get to see it from a different perspective.

"If we had sent her to the city by STARS it would have not helped as the family are all local. They would have had to travel into the city and then be told the same bad news." The charge nurse called and told me they are arriving right now and are in the quiet room. This way is harder for me as I will now need to sit them down with their family physician who is also coming and we will break the news the best we can. We will lay out the events and the current care and then we will inform them of the prognosis. We will soon need to extubate her after we have informed the family and let them say goodbye. I know that without a pressor and the breathing tube she will die right away. Sadly, she might pass away before we are ready to break the news and give them time to absorb it. All in all, this was the best outcome we could hope for with such a devastating prognosis. The real shock will be to the family members, I'm afraid.

I looked at Sarah and she felt as devastated as I felt, I'm sure. I had felt bad for I knew on arrival to the scene she must have had some really bad disease process inside attacking her body. We both had seen the home oxygen but unknown to us it had been set up the day before. I knew she was too young to be at home with oxygen and I had also thought it was odd, a silent warning to me you could say. The emergency physician said he compared the X-ray from today to one two weeks ago, and said it was a very aggressive spread of cancer. In addition, there was a big pleural effusion that had filled up her whole right lung over the last two weeks. He said he could possibly drain it with pleural tap now but then it would fill up right away. He then explained to us the hypotension was from a mechanical obstruction effect from the result of cancer and the fluid invading the lung fields. He looked at us with his most caring heart and told us both that we had done the right thing and thanked us for the excellent care. Then he went off to see some more pressing trouble and chaos in the ER. After all, it never stops. We both knew he would soon meet with the awaiting family and be giving them all the most tragic news a family can hear.

We just sat and finally Sarah said, "cancer sucks." I looked at her and said, "It's much, much worse than that, my friend. Let's get cleaned up and get out of here. I need a coffee and some fresh air." In no time, we were back in service and for the rest of the shift we were both exceptionally quiet. We needed time to understand our own feelings before we could or would talk to anyone else about them. That was part of the healing process despite the overwhelming feeling of losing or not being able to do enough. We all wanted to do as much as possible but sometimes that was not the right thing to do at all. Some days we were meant to lose and today was that day. At least we had the ability to keep her alive long enough for her family to say goodbye. I guess that should count for something. Well, if nothing else, it counted to us.

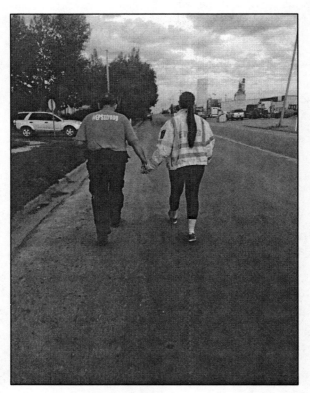

"Some days all we can do is walk away but
we need to walk away together"

Chapter 15: Tasting Death One More Time

"Bringing Them Back"

Almost getting killed a few separate times and seeing many people killed or dead made me realize just how very precious life is. We will never know how close we are to getting killed or hurt until it's too late. Well, unless our guardian angel protected us I would have to say. The day started just like any other day for Sarah and me. I had got Timmy's and our day was started right. No matter what happened, we would put up a good fight. We had no real plans for the next several shifts other than working on our approaches to dealing with our worst calls, helping each other with the grieving process as well and the debriefing process for our local service staff.

Every situation was so different and what works for one event won't work for others. The role of CISM was okay in theory but it was just one little part of the solution. We were going to try to help each other understand the different processes. It's a lifelong learning event, I'm afraid to say. Sarah also agreed with me on this huge part of EMS and health care. Nothing was guaranteed and nothing had always the same presentation or the same circumstances. Nothing we did was black and white. The EMS world had greyer parts than you could imagine or had more unclear events as we progressed throughout life it seemed. It helped our problem-solving ability but taxed our inner strength because it always causes inner turmoil just the same. You could not simply make a protocol to deal with everyday life events.

The best approach I knew for us was debriefing in small groups. We are not big into crowds with others we don't know after critical events or after certain calls. We all know sometimes the debriefing is therapeutic right after the call but sometimes people also need time. No two staff members are affected the same by any one event. The one thing that seemed to help was to show that we cared for each other and that we were always available to each other to listen, to be there and sometimes someone to hold us when we cry. The fact that we always had someone at our side was what mattered the most to me. I often thought back to some of the calls and wondered what or why life was the way it was.

Why was the pain and suffering so prevalent in this modern and sophisticated world? You would think with the current medication, diagnostic ability and treatment options we would be able to deal with the most common causes of pain. We should be able to lessen suffering better than we have been doing but it is not always the case. Our patients on the street are still abusing drugs in record numbers. The drugs are becoming stronger and the results of the street drug taken are reaching epidemic proportions but we just keep putting a Band-Aid on our social issues.

The one song that came to mind right then was "The Angel" by Sequoyah Rain. *"We are flying down the highways and got no time to kill and only the lord will know if we will win; it's a race against the clock, the golden hour is all he's got, there is a desperation in the cool night of wind; can't let that angel win again, stopped to grab a quick bite to eat and once again they are calling me she is tired of life and she took some pills"* is such a real part to me. One day many years ago we stopped three times throughout one-day shift to eat and every time we got another call. The last one was a train accident – we had one dead and three fighting to live. We tried our best that day but the angel of death ended up with three. We only got to keep one from the wrong side of heaven. The numbers had nothing to do with the effort; we put up one hell of a fight. We fought for every heartbeat, every ventilation and in the end fate won. We lost all but one.

Some days we will take anything the world throws at us and we make the best with what we can and that day it was one long and horrific call. It doesn't get any worse than that type of a call. Several years after that very tragic train versus a minivan call, we all lost my partner from that call in a very tragic event in a line of duty death. Darren was a gentle giant as an EMT and in the future, became an excellent paramedic. Then he became a tactical police officer with the Calgary Police Services but, tragically, he was shot in a training accident. The total sum of losses for that dreadful day just kept climbing in my mind. You can also add one ER nurse that was on that tragic day that later took her own life so the sum is greater than anyone can really ever know. That doesn't count the long-term effects on the train engineers, the first responders, the police officers that repeatedly see tragedy and for anyone else involved in working in EMS.

A little later that day I still could not get tragedy out of mind or my thoughts for I was just sitting and listening to another song and was struck how it showed me something I was feeling right about then. The lyrics from "Wrong Side of Heaven" by Five Finger Death Punch actually scared me, but nevertheless they were also true. The part that I really understood was *"Arms wide open, I stand alone, I'm no hero, and I'm not made of stone. Right or wrong, I can hardly tell. I'm on the wrong side of heaven and the righteous side of hell."* The wrong side of heaven and the righteous side of hell was all too often the road many EMS, police and many of our firefighters had traveled all in the line of duty. Many of us had to respond to or were dispatched or called out on the calls to go and try to help people or try and bring them back from hell, on too many occasions. That never even considered the hell any of our military members dealt with in the battles of a war zone. They were the ones I felt the sorriest for as they often came home broken and then were forgotten by our society.

Over the years, I lost count of the worst of the worst cases such as the murders, hangings, stabbings, beatings and, the child abuse events often with no consequences for the attackers or the guilty parties. The often runs of suicides were in threes. The tragic end of life was something we never got used to even if we dealt with it all to often. The only thing that made it something we could endure was the fact we had other people with us or around us that cared about each other. That's the only thing that brought us back from the darkness of evils' worst events. The sudden deaths along and the violent events are something we become hardened about in order to protect ourselves in many cases, I'm sure.

I had trouble understanding why some of our past co-workers as well as many of our patients would need to choose death over life as the only option left. What could be so bad that it was the only option they had left? It was my simple question without ever understanding the answer. Why people sought out death as the only solution to life or to staying alive for another day. A tragic waste of such a valuable life. I never understood how some people would come back with repeated overdoses and would live. Then the next one might be an unintentional event and they'd end up dead. Why were so many people constantly overdosing? By doing illegal drugs that it seems that they are always trying to get to a different place in time for the special high was strange to me. It's not worth the risk at all if you looked at it from an outsider's viewpoint.

The fact that people were killing themselves and causing so much self-harm tells me this world is not such a good place even if we often just see the good in our personal life away from our daily work. The good things were not as frequent in others' lives, I was sure. That was why some days I feel maybe hell is here on earth and heaven is just too far away to reach for so many of our patients. The calls that still bothered me are the hangings or violent deaths of the young and precious kids that haven't even had a chance to live yet. They are the ones that break my heart. That's not counting the kids killed in accidents or vehicle-related events. They are also bad but not as hard on the rescuers.

The pediatric calls are the ones that come back to haunt me when I never expect them. These calls make me question life, destiny, fate and living more than most of the calls I have seen or responded to in my career. Sadly, many people will never ever really feel comfortable talking to anyone about these types of call as they hurt too much, so they are just put on a shelf. This is likely why CISM doesn't lessen the effects or the incidents of PTSD in many EMS, police and firefighters. These are the calls that individual counselling should be used to help us all deal with when we are ready.

Looking back, these are the calls that would leave scars on my heart from side to side with the lucky ones we saved and the unlucky ones we lost. They will always haunt me even when the outcome was not as bad as it could have been. It was just another routine emergency call until we got to the scene then the call took a turn for the worse. Somehow, they all of a sudden became too real but I guess that was because they were real. The fact we repeatedly seen kids bleeding, crying, lying broken had many times marked our souls for life time of sleepless nights.

One day I was working a day shift and we were called for a breathing problem. It was not until we got close to scene that they updated the event – paediatric hanging. Then it became all too real in a second. Kids should not have to die this way. Families should not have to see the pain and know the suffering of losing a kid in such a traumatic and terrible way. We were often called for unknown problems or unknown situations only to find a disaster when we arrive.

We never had two calls the same but sometimes the calls had similar presentations. We would start off with our safety being the biggest priority and from then on it became an (A-B-C) check, which is simply an Airway – Breathing and Circulation approach if we thought they were awake or alive. But if we thought they were dead or unconscious we did a Circulation – Airway and then a Breathing check, which is now commonly referred to as (C-A-B) assessment. If we were not sure, we always got to the patient's side as quickly as possible and as we approached we could assess the patients from a distance. We would be looking for weapons, and signs of bleeding, distress or shock. Sometimes we were shocked to see signs of life when we didn't expect to and sometimes they were dead but looked as though they should still be alive.

As we pulled up we were met by a family member and I could tell they were scared. They were pleading for help. We never even thought or cared at that time about backup. We knew it would be coming if we needed it but it was also at least twenty-five to thirty minutes away. Thankfully we could use STARS but only if we had something to work with. Most days it was an asystole code and the outcomes were already predetermined.

Many overdoses, hangings and certain accidents cause tragic brain damage. Once the brain is without oxygen, without circulation and a buildup of CO_2 and lactic acid, it was always a losing outcome. Thankfully we understood and had practised aggressive airway and breathing management for years. We learned years later that was what saved brains although in many cases we did our best and never heard about the outcome. It was either a funeral in a week or one day you ran into a family member who told us the outcome. Most ended up in a city hospital on a ventilator and only time would tell the result. Very rarely we received a thank you card or the patient or family came and thanked us. When that happened, we felt like a million lives were won in the battle for life.

Sadly, we never knew the outcome in many cases and we were left wondering whether we did the right procedures or if we were wrong in our differential diagnosis. Many times, we were often guessing at the mechanism of injury and did not know the full history of events. Often, we would respond to a very bad event and find we had an unstable patient. We would get a pulse back in a cardiac arrest but not in time to save the brain. Often, we were not on scene fast enough to prevent permanent internal damage. We had good and bad outcomes. That was part of the job.

Sure, we had a pulse back and we were able to breathe for them and keep their BP up with pressors but they didn't wake up due to an anoxic brain event or brain damage not compatible with living. The only good outcome was if they could be an organ donor, which may sound horrific but after seeing death after death it was the only good outcome from such a waste of a life. It was the person's last effort to help someone else even if they could not help or would not be able to help themselves. Every day we tried to do a better job and as we provided better patient care the outcomes got better so then it was a constant challenge or battle to make them live; the reward was for them to be normal at the time their eventual discharge.

Today we entered the house with our kits and we were worried but not really sure what to expect. We walked into a young teenager who was just cut down from a small closet. Thankfully someone found her and cut her down right away. When I walked up I could see the ligature marks right away on her neck, which is a bad sign. I could also see the big eyes were open and she was looking at me so I felt a little better. I think my heart started to beat again. Sarah and I got to work. Oxygen with a NRB mask was applied; an IV was placed right away. The cardiac monitor was always applied immediately on any serious call and fortunately things were looking better and better by the minute. Our patient started to try to talk and her vital signs were improving. I called off the backup unit as I thought we would be okay. We applied a cervical collar just in case there was a spinal injury and then we applied her securely to a spinal board and with the family's help we moved her out to the unit.

Looking back, the house was immaculate. They were a loving, caring full house of family. Everyone was crying and upset. Everyone seemed to love her so much and couldn't understand. Why she had attempted to take her life? Was my question. This was so tragic. The police were on scene right away. In the end, we got the story and it was so sad. Just recently she was with another girl who had committed a crime; they were caught and she was charged as well. She came home and was so embarrassed that suicide was her way out. If she only knew she was still a kid and in the end not much would harm her. I'm sure this was out of character for her. We were fortunate that someone found her but then I realized we might easily have been too late. Just when we think we are okay, everything goes to hell. Our easy day just became a very bad day.

After getting her in the unit her breathing pattern changed and her breathing suddenly got much worse and irregular. I was so upset for not seeing that this was about to happen. I had called our backup unit off and I had thought we would be okay. Well fortunately for us the backup unit kept coming. I guess they thought they were going to be needed to cover our area so they were on scene in no time after I put out our distress call for backup. I wondered if they also knew something bad could happen and it was a pediatric hanging. They were caring EMS staff who had a special spot in their hearts for all kids. They didn't know how happy I was to see them suddenly come into the driveway while we were setting up to perform a Rapid Sequence Intubation (RSI). We had STARS dispatched right away but we were an hour away so we elected to secure an airway and get her stable, then we would meet them at a predetermined meeting location.

The police would escort us and make the landing zone safe just east of the overpass, which was a perfect spot to land a helicopter. In no time we had fire, police and our backup unit all at our side just waiting to help in any way possible. Today everyone knew it was a very serious call. Today it would not matter the race or the nationality for after all it was just a kid to everyone involved and that was all that should really matter.

In no time, we had her intubated and were trying our best to ventilate her faster than the normal rate to decrease the brain swelling. We ensured her blood sugar was okay as well. We carefully calculated her mean arterial pressure from her BP to ensure it was high enough to perfuse her delicate brain. We got one of the crew-members to drive and we were off as a convoy of EMS with a police escort. As soon as we crested the overpass STARS was on final approach for the landing. In seconds, the highway was closed by our RCMP, fire fighter escort and the chopper was on the ground right beside us. I was so thankful she was doing okay. Care was transferred over quickly, she was in STARS in minutes and they were off. The pilots simply lifted the BK-117 off the ground and at about fifty feet, dropped the nose and they were up and away. The miracles of flight will always amaze me. The pilots were the best in the world and we were fortunate to have them flying our many broken or unwell patients to a better place at speeds we could never replicate.

After they took off I just sat and wondered about the call from start to finish. I was so devastated that such an amazing, pretty little lady with everything to live for would attempt to take her own life. Looking down at her on our stretcher, she was an angel from heaven. Her race or her nationality would not have made any difference – she was a child and she would be special to everyone involved in her care. But even more, she was very like my daughter at that same age. She was someone's daughter. That was what hurt the most. Someone loved her very much. This little lady needed to live and we would give her every chance to come home when she out of harm's way and was ready for discharge.

I was so thankful how it turned out. Later on, that day, one of my friends with the STARS crew called me and told me to stop beating myself up as she did very well. They would leave her intubated for twenty-four hours and they expected a full recovery. That call lifted a huge weight off my chest. This one life we saved made up for the many losses we had recently seen. We needed that one specific call to show us we were in the right profession for the right reasons. We could not have asked for a better crew to back us up that day and seeing the STARS chopper on-final approach to land as we crested the overpass was like a miracle in the waiting. Sometimes angels come in all forms and from many events.

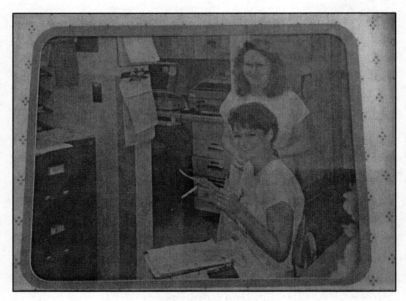

"Our Angels Never Let Us Down"

Chapter 16: Hitting the Wall

"No Place to Run"

The day will come when I look in the mirror and say no more. We responded to calls that don't faze you but one day you get back from another tragedy and say that's enough. There is no warning as to what will do it but happens all too often. The hardest thing I've seen is the parents after their loved one has been killed or taken their own life. The screams of pain are something I won't forget. The mangled remains after what a vehicle can do to a human body is unforgettable. One of the hardest things to me was the beatings or the violent murders. I can't imagine how people can do something so devastating to another human being and be able to walk away, think they didn't mean it or they're not guilty because of anger, drugs or alcohol. That reason doesn't cut it. Life should be sacred and precious. Today was one of those days when time will lessen the pain but it won't take it away. Some things are forever, our sacrifices for helping others, but then again it was still my job. That was the way it has to be.

Sarah was attending when we got called to clear up STAT. It was not very common but sometimes we went out of our way to help out. Today was one of those days. Ken was still riding third with us and that was okay, as we loved an extra pair of hands. Besides, it was our duty to help bring new members into our profession. We are being dispatched to back up the police at an assault. They need us now and can't wait for another service to arrive. We meet the nurses in the bay and transfer care. Becca is ready and we are out of the door in thirty seconds. All we know is that a child has been assaulted. En route we get an update, the scene is secure. I was driving and we were pushing the limits of our unit. The diesel was performing and the brakes were working extra hard in the corners although we were not slowing down much anyways. Today was going to be bad.

As we approached the scene the intersection was blocked by two police cruisers, we blew the intersection at maximum warp. We knew then this had to be really bad. Every police officer or RCMP available was helping. As we pulled up we had a plan. Sarah takes the monitor, I grab the airway and drug bag. Ken would take the trauma bag. We entered the scene and found the patient in the living room. The room was a huge bloody mess. There was blood on the walls and on the floor as well as all over the patient's body. It looked as though he'd been beaten with weapons such as bats or metal bars. The injuries were horrific. I went to the airway, Sarah was applying the monitor and Ken was helping grab airway equipment. I called for backup and fire was already en route. Today the next crew was not even close. STARS were also launched and they had a physician which was never a bad thing. They would come to the scene or the hospital as we required.

I had no idea what to do because the face was a swollen bloody mess with blood and bone deformity to the whole facial structure. I debated the next treatment but I was suddenly stopped. Sarah called out sinus bradycardia with a bounding pulse. Saturations less than 80% with crappy obstructed breathing, it's always bad. I shook my head and yelled, "Sarah I need help…" I grabbed the suction and yelled for a bougie. Sarah was grabbing the laryngoscope and the endotracheal tubes. I asked Ken to apply the high flow nasal prongs even though the face was a mess. I asked him to get ready to ventilate after I suction once. We needed it try to ventilate him but the airway was full of blood; likely teeth and a broken jaw, as well as every other bone in his face was broken. His eyes were already swollen shut which is a terrible sign. The portable suction was not great but I had no other options. The best suction was in the unit but that was not an option today.

We were surrounded by a group of police and suddenly the fire crews walked in. I asked a few of them to try and get IVs, a scoop and we needed a landing site as close as possible. I told the captain we were in big trouble. Until we got an airway, we were doomed. He understood and had seen this before. I'm sure he was praying for us all. Today we had the airway from hell. The other very tragic thing was it was someone's child. It was somebody who didn't deserve this. Nobody in the world deserved this.

The airway was not getting better. I could not suction very well. We were getting big clots and had some teeth broken in the mouth and at the back of the throat. I was trying to get them out with the Magill forceps. I asked Sarah to try and pass the smaller endotracheal tube as I suctioned and tried to place the bougie past the blood. I was guessing by landmarks but it was a terrible approach and no one's fault. It was a three-person technique. Ken was applying the Sellick manoeuvre but it was not very effective because the jaw was broken and the swelling and bleeding were not helping us. I found a little opening and pushed the tube through the blood and the clots while trying to suction but not effectively. Sarah passed the tube and I reached to the outer structure of the trachea. I felt the endotracheal tube pass by the vocal chords. It was a miracle. We had an airway. Next the cuff was inflated and we attempted to ventilate. As expected the chest was also broken internally. This kid was so broken. No one did this accidentally – this was a vicious and horrific attack.

The chest was rising but only on the left and not the right side. I percussed the chest and as I suspected, a pneumothorax as well as a hemothorax was most likely. I grabbed a 14-gauge needle and inserted it over the third midclavicular rib on the right side. We decompressed it right away to prevent problems down the road, or today in the air. The ETCO2 was registering as high as 65 mmHg so we had to get ventilating. The Sp02 was as low as 60% before we got an airway and the Sp02 was rising but not as fast as I hoped for. We needed to get the oxygen to the brain and get the ETCO2 down to around 32–35 mmHg with the LP-15 as our guide. Finally, we had an airway. Next, we had to worry about the circulation as well as the rest of the examination, which had not been done yet.

Then we had to evaluate our required treatments and ensure we could do our best in the time we had. We needed to know the full impact of the trauma on the patient so that we could perform the right treatments. Normally the patient assessment would have been done but an airway emergency is one of the really bad things that can interrupt any primary survey other than a safety issue or a cardiac arrest. Sarah took over ventilating. The first IV was in and the second was also in thanks to our fire staff. Thankfully they are trained EMR and EMTs on the service. Technically they are not our staff but in emergencies we do our best. It has always been one of my rules: "Do what it takes to save a life."

The first BP was 220/134 which is terrible. We had to get the ETCO2 down right now, get the oxygen saturations over 90% and keep them there. I raised the head of the patient about ten degrees while Sarah ventilated. We suctioned the endotracheal tube to remove about 100 mLs of blood out of the deep tracheal areas. The oxygen saturations started to rise soon after. The oral gastric tube was inserted carefully and blood was removed from the stomach as well as considerable amounts of air, which was most likely from our forcefully ventilating prior to the intubation attempt.

I patched directly to the STARS and OLMC and thankfully I got permission for Mannitol which is not usually used before a head CT but today we would take our chances. I got a Foley catheter in and it was draining right away. There was not much else we could do. The STARS doctor asked about the weight and as he was over fifty kilograms approximately, he asked us to administer 1 gram of

Tranexamic acid (TXA) over ten to twenty minutes. It was started even though it's not used as commonly in children. Today we would try everything possible. We needed a miracle but we all knew the miracle had already been denied as evil overcame the day. The RCMP in charge of the scene stated to us as he walked past that it was a home invasion. They had three other young adults in custody. The fire chief said they had a landing zone one block away right beside the school. Ironically, it was spring break or the kids involved would have been in school, one would hope.

The next step was to move to the unit and then we would move over to the school. The next BP was much better but still high at 170/110 so I elected to give a little Versed 2.5 mg IV and Fentanyl 50 mcg slow IV just to ensure the child was relaxed. The heart rate had come up to 75 bpm, which was a better sign. The ETCO2 was better and we were ventilating one every four seconds and Sarah was happy with the Sp02. The decompression needle was still letting air out and some blood but not bad.

The head to toe exam was tragic, most likely multiple skull fractures, facial fractures, and the right chest had the worst of the injuries. There would be other not so obvious injuries. The pediatric trauma team would ensure he had the best chance possible. Most likely the neurosurgical service would have to intervene ASAP to lessen the brain damage if possible. Only time would tell. I looked at everyone and said we have done a good job and meant it. I was dripping sweat from my forehead. Sarah, Ken, and I high-fived each other at the same time. Despite the tragic call, we had done our best and we'd got an airway when it looked impossible. We had just moved into the unit when we heard the STARS chopper overhead. They would be down and waiting for us as we travelled the block and parked by the ball diamonds.

We had an RCMP officer staying with the child and he would follow him through to the trauma team and admission process. Despite the terrible events, we all worked so well together as a team. We had the right firefighters today as both went right to work and got us IVs as we were busy trying to get the airway secure. That was what teamwork was all about. The RCMP I noticed were strategically placed at every doorway. After a quick thought, I understood it was a methodical approach to protect us. They never get the true appreciation they deserve from all our EMS staff but they deserved it. When we worked as a team we make our personal image better in my eyes. We had to remember that many of the police and firefighters also had kids at home. These calls are hard on us but just as difficult for them. No one is immune to the effects of trauma, death and the many tragic events we see while trying to help others in need.

We met the STARS crew as we pulled into the ball field. The STARS crew jumped in took a look at the mess and they too were shocked. I told them in simple words, "It was an airway from hell. It took three of us to get the tube in." We told them about the bad BP, the initial low saturations and the high ETCO2. All of this would need to be relayed to the trauma team. They also checked the head to toe exam and were concerned about the right chest injuries. The STARS doc asked his crew to initiate the blood products in the air as the Hgb was low. The lactate was over ten, which is terrible but expected in bad situations. In no time, the patient was transferred over and they were loading and ready to take off. We moved back and watched them warm up and get ready to leave. After the warm up we could hear the sounds from the helicopter change, the pitch of the rotors changes and lift off was achieved. In no time, they were climbing and circling towards the destination hospital. We all watched the chopper until it was out of sight.

Every one of us was praying. I'm sure the outcome would be better than it looked but we all knew, even Ken, that this was very bad. After the X-rays and the CTs and the neurological examination the real story would be known. But most likely the outcome would not be known for a day or two until they could decide whether the brain had a chance. Then we slowly went to the unit. I started to do the ePCR but said, "Coffee and let's take a break, and then we can start this clean up." We went to the base and got a supervisor to get us coffee. We let dispatch know we would be out of service for several hours so they could flex us some relief. Today we'd earned our break. Thankfully, Ken was with us today, as well as the firefighters who were so helpful. A second ALS team would have been really good but we made it work. We made our stand and we fought one very hard and an intense battle to save a life. Nobody can take that away from us. Yes, we may have deviated from protocols and not done it the textbook way, but we saved a life.

We got to the base and another crew came out and met us that had also just returned from a transfer. They were volunteering to help clean and restock. I said, "Let's do this really quickly and then we can work on the ePCR." We needed to go to the police station for statements and there was a debriefing at the end of shift. It is set up at the end of all our shift. Then we could actually let our protective walls down and be open and be honest about our feelings. The volunteer Fire fighters involved will be invited to attend as well. I was okay to go but somewhat not looking forward to the debriefing. Kids suck but this was worse. Greg, Ken, as well as Derrick were out helping redo our kits. Refresh our medication kits, then we restocked all airway equipment and finally our IV supply stock. That's when I realized our volunteer fire had put in a 16 gauge and a 14 gauge. That was amazing. Looking back to how the fire and police had made our whole call flow made me proud. God, it was so good to have backup that worked as a team and not one time had we had a disagreement or a bad word about any interactions.

We had the other unit join us with coffee and some "Birthday Cake Timbits." Heather and Dave were our relief crew and they came in early for us. They had our backs and always would. We would do the same thing for them. They both came up and gave us both a big hug for they had heard about our bad pediatric call. No matter how bad some of the calls were, we are supported by our EMS family. It was my only real family that knew my pain and saw me on my worst days. Thankfully, several of the hospital staff were some of my biggest supports over the years. The doctors were as well; even though they never said as much, we knew they were part of our team. Most of them understood our battles and appreciated our efforts. We all had one rule after every call. We thanked them even if they were having a bad day and we were always honest with them.

They would always have our backs as long as we were honest with them and we treated our patients as people. That was easy in my way of thinking for it was our job. A few times over my career I had missed or not done certain normal things and if you didn't do it, just say you didn't. The few times I made a medication error I said right up front what and why I did something. In the end, it worked out okay, but a few times I was terrified. Just the fact I had made an error was enough to give me a bad day. I was always so thankful that we had a good working arrangement with the ER and hospital staff; over the years they did their best for us.

After the call, we got to the debriefing at the local RCMP detachment. We were always treated with respect and we knew they appreciated us but after all, it was mutually deserved for we helped and respected each other. We met in a big room with coffee and refreshments. The on-call chaplain was there and there were a few staff members from victim services. About eight firefighters arrived and I was praying they would have no calls until it was over. They had earned the rest. After a short informal introduction was done around the room of all attending, everyone felt part of the group. A prayer was said over us all which was not common but not one head was up. Respect was given despite the different cultural beliefs I'm sure, that can come from a room of multiple rescuers. Then we were ready to start what was going to be an intense but therapeutic session. It started with a really good and honest reminder we are here today for CISM support and this is not considered punitive nor are there any discipline concerns that will be addressed. The purpose is sharing our version of the events, how we participated and what our roles were. We were reminded that our feelings were real and we would not be abandoned. If we needed support it would be provided.

We were reminded today that many people went above and beyond their duty to help save a life. We worked as a team and we did our best. It was not a normal situation and the scene as well as the different parts of today will affect us all differently. We should know the efforts to save someone so traumatically injured affect us all differently and at different times. Over the days to come we may have days when we feel overcome with grief or sadness and at any time we should seek support through the peer support set up for all of us. The one part that was brought up by someone with a lot of experience said, "that no matter how we deal with the event today it takes time to recover from traumatic exposure." Pain is pain and we must know the pain to know we are alive. Sometimes it's that pain that helps us keep going.

The one part I liked after attending the debriefing was the approach to "psychological first aid." The effect comes from the group helping to empower and inform the members of the group to open up, to enhance their ability to deal with the stressful event, and to help build them back up so that after they walk out the doors they are ready for the next encounter. We get knocked down individually or as a group but together we can help each other up. Together we can ensure people are not left behind. I love that analogy: *"If we get knocked down seven times in life we get back up eight times."* Sometimes we need our friends or our co-workers to get us back up and there is no shame in that.

We are human, we feel pain, we see suffering and we all know it is wrong. That is part of what makes the turmoil inside our hearts. Sometimes the biggest and hardest people are affected the most.

We all have hearts and we all have feelings. Anyone in our profession can be broken into pieces whether you are careful or not. You can't be unaffected from the events and the calls we must face and encounter. We come and make the best out of the worst of the situations possible and then after we go home they are not over yet. They still live inside us. It's how we deal with them that will make us a fighter and with the help of others we can overcome the negative effects.

After the rounds of debriefing I learned to appreciate one important lesson. We are all human. The new and senior members are just as affected by the events we see from time to time. We need to ensure for the rest of our career we are our partners' backup. We need to be an emotional crutch someday. We need to recognize the effects of being overcome with stress and know we must intervene from time to time to save the life of our friends. The "Superman Song" from the band the Crash Test Dummies has two separate parts that say so much to me as an EMS professional and hospital staff member co-workers. The chorus is so moving and describes the despair and destruction we see from time to time. No matter what events or situations we respond to we will always do our best and face every call or event as a team. ***This part is so true to me.***

> *Superman never made any money*
> *For saving the world from Solomon Grundy*
> *And sometimes I despair the world will never see*
> *Another man like him.*

I think of this after our call and after coming back home after the call.

> *Hey Bob, Supe had a straight job*
> *Even though he could have smashed through*
> *any bank*
> *In the United States, he had the strength, but he*
> *would not*

Folks said his family were all dead
Their planet crumbled but Superman, he
forced himself
To carry on, forget Krypton, and keep going.
Tarzan was king of the jungle and lord over all
the apes
But he could hardly string together four words: "I
Tarzan, You Jane."
Sometimes when Supe was stopping crimes
I'll bet that he was tempted to just quit and turn
his back
On man, join Tarzan in the forest
But he stayed in the city, and kept on
changing clothes
In dirty old phone booths till his work
was through
And nothing to do but go on home.

The End of Our Days Thoughts…

Just know when you go home you are not alone. Don't be afraid to call a friend and if it means they see you cry then that is okay. They will see and know you're more than Superman. You're human and you care too much. But all the same you matter. I want to share something I came across that describes words from the heart. Thank you for sharing this with the world.

> *"Grief is like the ocean; it comes on waves ebbing*
> *and flowing. Sometimes the water is calm, and*
> *sometimes it is overwhelming. All we can do is learn*
> *to swim."*

> –Vicki Harrison

"Making it Right"

One of the biggest challenges we face today is to foster our profession into a better world. It maybe sounds easy but it's far from it. Imagine us as being the new kids on the block of life. We have to sustain ourselves, we need to grow, we need to adapt, and we need to master our skills. All while trying to prove we deserve the right to be part of the team. With the past structure or set up, we were under medical guidelines which had some flexibility. Then we lowered the bar and we were lazy when it came to ensure we increased our professional responsibilities, so we were put under protocols. Over time, we got lazy and we provided sub-standard care. The physician group that overlooked our profession stepped in and took over for obvious reasons. We made the errors and we were not accountable for them under the old Health Disciplines Act (HDA). We messed up, in my eyes, I would suggest.

The protocols became stricter and then came On Line Medical Control commonly referred to as OLMC. We dug our own grave to limiting our medications and our standard skills and we required guidance to perform our normal job more and more. We needed to ensure we always assessed our patients properly, learn our patients' conditions, treat our patients as though they matter and we need to be 110% accountable for our actions. I support OLMC 110% but more as a consulting process rather than part of a protocol. We need to increase our education at all levels. We need to practise and become more proficient in all skills; we need to be the master of them all and not just a few of them. When we are asked to assist other professional bodies, we need to ensure we display respect and never try to lessen another's work to make us look superior at any time. Now we have finally entered the Health Professions Act (HPA) we can take ownership of our past disasters and raise the bar. We can become accountable to each other and our profession. Better yet, we can be accountable to our patients and to our needs within society today.

Somehow, we forgot why we became paramedics and instead became servants of the greater health care system. I sat back and said we need to change this and somehow, we will. This was my main mission before I walked away from the disaster we all walked into without a back door. We had to get out or we were all doomed to suffer under a system of control. I would make a back door and get others to follow. We would escape a sinking ship and rebuild a system where EMS would be the elite system it should be. We needed common sense to prevail and we needed to build wisdom into our current EMS system. Our education needed to consist of degrees (degree in EMS), then the master's (master's in EMS), and then a doctorate (Ph.D. in EMS). The education and training structure needed to be significantly enhanced for our profession to succeed and survive.

Over the next several days I would draft my idea and get Sarah, Ken and Robin to break it apart and find holes in it. I would make the document stronger and better. Somehow, we could and would influence the people leading our profession or at least give them some ideas or solutions. When it was ready I would forward it to the people who could and would influence the EMS world for a better future. I have attached an idea for change. It's just an idea and it's my idea so I own it. 110%. As with all ideas it will have merit and I will have flaws. If nothing else, it's food for thought for our future.

This was my own personal idea to change our profession just from looking at our system and thinking how can we make it better. The challenge is in the hands of our professional members. The next step is all yours, my friends.

Professional Transitional Requirements
for
The Emergency Medical Services

Dales Idea: Implementation by 2019

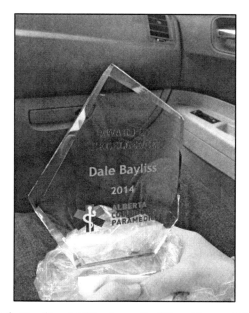

Dale Bayliss ACP - Award of Excellence 2014

Over the last several years, I've been looking ahead contemplating the future of EMS as a profession. Trying to think how we can improve our future. We need to take our profession to the next level. The next level is from our current status to somewhere around a world of excellence. We need to push the current limits of our practice but first thing's first, we need to not only exceed the minimum of the current education status but we need to push the boundaries. We need to create our Emergency Medical System (EMS) as the leaders in the health care around the world.

Our EMS world needs us to function at an optimal level, despite the limitations enforced on us by the current emergency medical culture. If we continue to be followers, we will lose our identity. If we don't fix our broken system and make some global changes, we are doomed before we even get truly started. It's time for people to be proud of who and what we are as a profession. Let's make tomorrow an EMS system that is second to none. Let's be winners as well as leaders in our profession. Let's work for a unified change to be the members' people count on 24/7.

Now just imagine this as an idea. I would say to you all we should never limit our "Imagination for Positive Change." This is my idea and I will own it but more importantly I will share my vision with my EMS world of the changes we need for a positive and productive future. We can all look at our present situation and make our future more positive and enhance a unique change for our future. Imagine a world of EMS excellence, and then let's just make it happen. I want to leave this profession knowing I have made a difference and nothing else will do. When I'm successful, then my mission is also successful. Only then can I walk away knowing it was worth the personal sacrifices and the long sleepless nights. Only then will I know my EMS family are going to be safe and have a future in health care.

Let's remove or eliminate the preceptor mentality. Let us start to mentor our newest members into the profession. We are all learning and expanding our horizons as a group of one. Let's make all of us accountable for improving our profession that ensures we are lifted to the highest level of being leaders in the health care systems, community practitioners and thus educators of our community's health emergency medical care systems. We are not considered Basic Life Support (BLS) or Advanced Life Support (ALS) we are now considered a Health Care System and it's a continuum of care from the start of a 9-1-1 call to arrival at the local ER or critical care centre. Everyone is part of our care and it's not us against him or her at or with any EMS service. All fire, police and EMS are considered equals and treated with mutual respect.

Let's move our profession into the twenty-first century. If you want to see just how well we can go as a profession. You just need to look at what our EMS colleagues are doing in other countries. We should aim to try and exceed or provide the equivalent to what is available. In one example in Europe who even in 2016 are working with the critical care centres to provide critical care interventions or procedures, in rural or urban centres or while responding to or with emergency medical services calls.

The greatest example I can provide is that our EMS members are actually performing interventional radiology procedures at accident scenes to slow down serious internal bleeding. They are also mandated to perform 12-leads and treat heart attacks without OLMC. They are accountable to be leaders in the emergency medical care world. They are the ones we should be trying to replicate, if I was in control or had a chance to change our direction of care. Let's dream for the moon and take what we achieve as a start and just keep trying to enhance our EMS world from within. We need to at least meet the standard of care but we can exceed the National Occupational Competencies of Paramedics Level (NOCP's) in time. We can be a leader in the future of EMS care just as we were in the past with some hard work, increased effort and the willingness to see change.

We need to exceed the minimum level of care across Canada. The standards must be set, maintained and enforced. We can't just think we deserve our status as health care professionals; we must deserve our right and treat it as a privilege. Nothing in education or health care should be taken for granted. We are the professionals under a credence are the catalyst to make the right change. We must ensure our profession enhances the educational and professional changes and guides our profession to be the best of the best. Without our growth, we will not survive. Without our complete and willing participation, our profession is going to be annihilated. We can't survive the traditional process without positive and organized change.

Just think that being positive will enable us all and then think we "finally have a vision and a specific purpose as a profession." I will put out the idea for the change and you, my friends, will make it happen even if I can't be part of the change. Several of you will chuckle and see through this as "Dales Way", but secretly it's part of Tim's Way, Cheryl's Way, Len's Way, or even Heather's Way. So yes, my friends, we all have people we respect highly, learn from, even if we don't always see or follow them on their pathways of life. We will take the best from people and use it to enhance our world if we want to excel for the right reasons, I would think.

As Abraham Lincoln said many years ago, but is most appropriate today: *"Determine that the thing can and shall be done, then find the way."* The next step is realizing the changes we need to make and then make it happen. The reasons are laid out in the following paragraphs and I leave the rest up to our EMS family members to make it happen at the cost of change.

The first part was easy. Let's fix the educational institutions' requirements to be accountable for our students as they are our EMS members after they enrol. The example I will use is the educational institutes in Alberta are all controlled directly by direction from the Alberta College of Paramedics (ACP) who have now made it possible to advance our levels of proficiency and knowledge. Emergency Medical Responders (EMRs) are treated like they should be as solely ready for entrance into the profession. The Primary Care Paramedics (PCPs) then take it to the next level of mastering BLS skills and are seeing entrance towards traditional ALS skills and wisdom. The Advanced Care Paramedics (ACP) members are the experts in any Advanced Life Support (ALS) skills. Finally, the Critical Care Paramedics (CCPs') are leaders and educators within the profession. The days of enforcing the unrealistic scenario testing are long gone.

The initial EMRs are starting with a wider scope as they now have a sixteen-week program. They must not only be proficient, but also confident in the required skills. The days of teaching students only how to pass a scenario are long gone. Students are using high fidelity testing at all levels including increased clinical exposure. The schools won't be allowed to put students through with a minimum skill level. The days of two or fifteen intubations are not acceptable. The more we can see and learn within a learning environment is mandatory, along with high fidelity simulation we can ensure the graduates are ready to function as entry to practice at the level they have achieved.

Students are taught the one way, which is the right way recognizing we will have constant changes in education just as medicine and emergency care is constantly being improved. This is very like the past medical school's structure. Schools must teach towards a standard curriculum and not just enough to pass a test. We should not limit education but expand it across all areas. The educational requirements must be geared to a more rounded education.

The initial courses in EMS education are not providing competence, they are ensuring base knowledge. The EMR testing is reflective of that in they must achieve a minimum grade to pass the institutional requirements. With the increased practicum hour requirements of hospital, ambulance and community placements, the students are not just "pushed through," but are mentored. It's also required for all students to pass a five-day driving course in the EMR course; at the PCP level, the driving course is even more aggressive and appropriate for driving an emergency vehicle of all sizes and configurations.

Participation is mandatory in all components. It's essentially an introduction to patient care at the EMR level. You can't be tested on imaginary or unrealistic scenarios as that's not a logical or recognized component in a leading professional body. Then at the PCP level the training is more advanced with courses such as ACLS, PALS, NRP and many other courses to ensure they are ready for critical care participation with all ACP and critical care members are mandatory. Members can and will slowly increase personal knowledge and reach achievable goals, all while continuing to help our profession evolve. We all are accountable for our success.

Let's expand our Advanced Care Paramedics (ACPs) to use additional pharmacology or pharmacological components to become qualified to work as an equivalent in the current emergency rooms as staff or co-workers. Then let's expand the critical care members' scope and increase the pharmacology agents available to them to perform as masters at the critical care level. They need the equipment, the knowledge, the wisdom and the ability to be leaders in the profession. They will be our in-house educators for their fellow co-workers as well. They too are selected to be mentors, educators and leaders to all other allied healthcare professionals.

We all need to be advocates of the profession at work and also out in the communities. We will need to work with the educational institutions to continue to be leaders in the profession as we grow and expand our scope of practice. They all will be our future leaders and role models for the profession. We need our members placed strategically throughout our communities to enhance health care and to ensure our profession is the vision of leadership and not a servant of a stagnant health care system.

Critical care is the optimal care and Basic Life Support (BLS) is a standard for all patients, so why should we settle for only BLS. For example, when you go to the ER you don't only see the nurses but you are guaranteed to see the physician as well. So why in the real world do we limit citizens to only BLS care, when they deserve Advanced Life Support (ALS) capabilities on all calls.

For all levels of care, if you can justify your actions it was an appropriate intervention. For example, if you were to do a 12-lead ECG on a patient who only required a 3-lead, that should not be faulted and the equipment should remain on during transport. It is always beneficial to monitor your patients. When you think about it EMRs can and should be able to use end tidal CO_2 monitoring just as PCP should be expected to perform and interpret basic 12-leads in the real world. Just think about it, our monitors are worth up to $30,000 so let's use them to their fullest potential. Just the fact the LP 12 or LP 15 monitors will do ST segment monitoring is reason enough to leave a 12-lead system attached during transport.

We should be able to positively change our profession and not just sit back and ignore the inadequacy of a system that has need of additional structure or an enhanced functionality. Most errors in a profession are system errors. Therefore, let's change the profession and not attack the practitioners. Let's ensure we achieve a mastery of our profession and become equals in the profession and not followers. You can't save lives as a follower. You can't lead from the bottom. You become a leader with dedication, endurance and determination and you must be able to adapt to change as our dynamic system changes. Which truly demonstrate that our evolutionary existence is justified. Otherwise we become obsolete and our profession becomes assimilated by our allied health workers to enhance their own existence.

I've been reflecting too, on the day I received the 2014 Paramedic Award of Excellence. I must uphold the belief and confidence of the people who nominated me in my ability to be a leader or a member providing the requirements to receive the Award of Excellence. We need to strive to improve our profession at all levels. We need to enhance the profession in a positive way, even if I don't believe in the current structure of education or evolution of our profession. Until my dying day, I will not let my profession down. I will always help my friends in times of need. I will not forsake the people who demonstrated their support for my passion for EMS and our patients. As professionals, we should be able to learn from our errors and be accountable to our members and to ourselves.

Dale M Bayliss RN/EMT-P/ACN

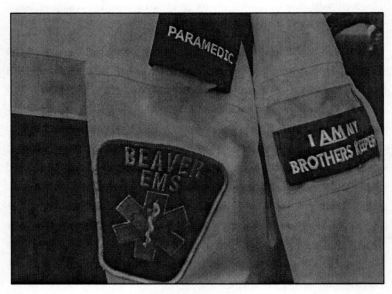

"My EMS Team Matters"

"Making True Friends for Life"

The only reason we can be able to survive in the EMS world, I think is due to our partners. We can help so many people but we need the right partners. If we had the right partners we could help anyone in almost any situation. I would call it a synergistic effect. At times, we would have faced even worse calls than normal but by having the right partner it made the call manageable. We could face the most severe trauma case or a very unstable medical patient and the effects of the teamwork would increase our success rate tenfold.

My whole life, what has saved me and helped my patients the most was a partner that sometimes was even much better than me. When we worked together we could see and do twice as much. When you face any problem from two angles your success is 150% better in almost all circumstances. Yes, I will be the first to admit it that there were times my EMT's saved me more than I can ever count. They would see things I missed and together we made the patient's life a little better. We always managed to get each other through the easy, the routine and the roughest of calls.

During the initial calls, it was my partner showing me the ropes from call to call. From that first day on, it was clear to me we all had a part in every call as a team. With every call, we each had a different perspective, as well as, each having a unique picture from a different view every time. When we put our pictures together we made our call, determining priorities and then we would make a plan of attack. On one call, I would perform the vital signs and my partner would assess the patient. On the next, we would switch. As we progressed in the profession we assumed more and more skills. We mastered our skills and then we taught them to our students or mentored our new partners.

We knew each other's strengths and weaknesses. Many times, I would let my partner attempt a skill and if they needed help they would just ask. In the ALS world when I had an EMT partner I would have more responsibility. I never thought I was better than they were – I just had a different set of skills. For example, if we had a bad call that needed ALS airway skills I would manage the airway while my partner started the IVs and then they would apply the monitor. But many days we would multitask and get things done, as they were needed, as a team of one. We would not be told we could just do the job.

Many times, if we had a paramedic student working with us I would give them first attempt at the advanced airway procedures such as an intubation and if they had trouble I would take over. Thinking back to our recent call with an airway from hell it was everyone working to get the job done. It would sometimes take two to four of us to get the airway and then we all could breathe a little more easily. Rules or guidelines were suggestions but at the end of the day we did our job together. I was still responsible for any ALS skills or procedures but we would do any skill or procedure together. That was the way it was in my unit. I never disregarded a suggestion from my partner unless it was one to cancel on scene, which I would not do unless it was a simple fall or a trivial event.

Too many times I'd seen this turn out badly for patients and for the crew. I had seen several crews try to cancel on as many as calls as possible, or neglect to use their stretcher or to even assess their patients. A good rule of thumb that it is easy to apply your monitor, start an IV or put in a heparin lock on any unknown condition. Sometimes by applying a little oxygen you made everyone feel much better and it causes no harm. They were easy treatments to justify, as they often proved useful in the end.

Not every crew had it that lucky. Every once in awhile, I'd come across the paramedic or EMT partners from hell. Ones that are rude, condescending or just plain stupid, when it came to teamwork. That was not the worst part; it was when they didn't want to help people that was the most painful thing. Those were the people I wished were working as a plumber or something else. I wanted and would only work with people I trusted and with staff that wanted to be there. On the odd day, I would get stuck with someone else because my regular partner was off but on the whole, I couldn't complain. My last two partners had been to hell and back with me. I would not have made the trip without them back safe and still alive. I owe them both my life. I always wondered how or who arranged our partners but somehow, we mastered our calls and we made the EMS team as well as it could be if it was at all possible.

The best thing about being with someone you liked working with was that you could share the workload and the responsibility; also, you could bounce your ideas off each other without feeling embarrassed or intimidated. The workload some days was a little heavy and when you got tired you could switch out or if you needed a day to drive or a day to attend, it all worked out in the end. Some days I was actually too tired to drive so I would have to attend. Our safety was a mutual responsibility. We looked after each other in ways that kept us both safe. When someone was not nice to my partner I would automatically try to attend. When I was ready to sedate my patient on a bad day my partner took over until they crossed the line and then anything was possible from extra medications, to four-point restraints or to jail.

The most unique part of a good partner was the extra stamina it provided when we needed it the most. We work long hard shifts on many days. With the right partner, we borrow positive energy on our bad days. It just amazes me how much a smile or an offer to help make our days so much easier. When we are awakened for a 02:00 a.m. call and we can't see straight or we are just not awake yet, it can be our partner's push and encouragement that helps us get rolling, figure out where we are going and ensure we get to the scene safely. Then when we are not really mentally alert or not at our best, our partner always has our back and ensures we are safe. Both Lisa and Sarah had protected me more than once, just as I had saved them from harm a time or two. One time I had come up from the side as my partner was being attacked. I had hit the attacker at a dead run. Then I used a good hockey check and took them out against a trauma room door. I picked them up and carried them outside and we had our own dispute until a few big police officers came with lights and sirens as our backup and then his day was over. The fight against three of us was a lose-lose for the bad guy. At least my partner was safe and the blood on the floor that day was only partly mine.

One of the special traits of a good EMS partner is openness. I would say what makes our team so good is the fact we are willing to be vulnerable with each other. Although I was the paramedic and they were the EMT I would share my thoughts and ideas. Or if I was heading down the wrong road my partner could easily turn me around and point me in the right direction. I would tell Sarah my weaknesses and I would be honest in every situation. If I had my doubts or was unsure about life or my problems I would share them without any chance of being criticized. I went into every call with my partner with my guard down and undefended, for I trusted them. I was so much more successful if we went in as a team. But at the end of the day we came out as a team.

The biggest thing that made our team always work was we had honesty and integrity with each other and to the people we worked with. Our valuables were always safe with each other. I would know her PIN and she would know my PIN for our debt and credit cards. We shopped for each other and we also watched each other's stuff and made sure our stuff was always safe. The only time I crossed the line was when I stuck an extra twenty in her purse for our coffee or gave her an extra Timmy's card when she wasn't looking. It was my own way of making her smile from time to time.

One event I had was after we'd had several bad calls and at the end of our shift I went home in a bad way. I had a really bad day and my night was worse. I texted my partner and made sure she was okay later that night. She said she was okay and I hung up after a short discussion. She knew my day was bad for in less than ten minutes she was at my door and one look at her told me she was worried. The offer of a coffee was a good idea as sleep was not right at that time. In a few minutes, we were off for a coffee and we had each other to share our pain and ensure we each had someone to talk to. That was something I needed more than anything. Even if it was in the middle of the night we had our own debriefing in our own style. Our small debriefings worked better. We had so much more comfort knowing we both could count on each other without regrets or reservations and to talk to each other about anything that needed to be discussed. It was never uncomfortable; even if it was painful, once it was out we felt better.

Somehow, she had known the calls were extra hard for me and she gave me the time; and when I reached out she knew I was having a bad day. It was not an unusual day but somehow the calls just all had a bad outcome. One patient was full of cancer and on her last few days but was fighting to live as long as possible. The part of dying from being short of breath was never easy to watch. There was not enough oxygen in the end to sustain her relatively short life. The other one was a cardiac arrest of a younger gentleman who had just collapsed at home with some younger children present. It was so tragic to see the kids crying for daddy and a wife in pure shock. It was just a bad few calls and somehow, they were draining. The RCMP was so helpful as well and the victim services were miracle workers for in terms of support. Looking back, it was still a winning team despite a lost battle for a human life.

Sometimes we need to take the initiative and reach out to our partners after the bad and the good calls just to make sure we are doing okay, even if we feel it's an uncomfortable question. Even after a good call we can beat ourselves up. My best example is if we miss a few intravenous catheter insertions (IV's) in a row. We challenge ourselves to give one hundred and ten percent but even the best of the best can make mistakes or have trouble handling a difficult call. I think sometimes we miss the easy ones to prove we are human and never perfect. I've done really hard IVs and missed, and I've done really easy IVs and missed.

I've prayed to God to help me get an IV in a life and death event and I was successful despite the outcome in the end for the patient's life. At the time, the only thing that mattered was for me to get the IV in on the first attempt. Even if we lost the battle for human life we got the IV and with the IV we did our best so there are many ways to look at our performance. I learned to help my partners and I would praise them despite the outcome. I would smile and say missing an IV keeps us honest. I would try to teach others to praise the good attempts and praise my partners for the missed attempts and help them get it on the second attempt. When they struck out it was my show and even then, I'd miss sometimes but not very often.

In many ways, we were our own biggest and worst critics on ourselves. We wanted to always do a better job and even if it was not a threatening or stressful call we tried to be as good as possible. Babe Ruth had a good quote. It simply said: *"You just can't beat the person that never gives up."* Well I guess in many ways when it came to starting IVs you needed that attitude; the rest was just simply technique.

Thinking back to what made the winning team in EMS was by starting off on the right foot. The one part that built our winning team or our partnership the first time we met was our respect for each other, despite our different levels of education. The respect to trust each other and we both knew we could and would say or ask anything of each other without feeling bad. As a really good example, I would sometimes look at an Electrocardiogram (EKG) and then show Sarah just in case I was missing something. We would debate strange readings and a few times she caught me on something I should have seen right away such as the miniature pacing spike or a strange pattern in aVR on a 12 lead ECG which can be indicative of a left main coronary artery occlusion (LMCA) or severe triple vessel disease or also called (3VD) in many cardiac research papers. So even if she was an EMT we were a ALS team. What I missed she picked up and what she missed I picked up and that was the way it should be as a team.

The other part was the mutual respect we had for others in uniform. The level of respect was also part of the code of honour. The best example I can think of is we respect others in uniform no matter what the uniform – it's something we are accustomed to do as we were brought up I would think in most places and to anyone in uniform like that. When we were kids we were taught the RCMP were always to be respected and we would not harm or ever put them in danger for any reason. If I was to tell a police officer off or even think of it as a teenager my dad would've killed me. Dad also was very clear: "If you ever do drugs I will kill you." Thankfully he never condemned drinking in moderation. So even my dad demanded a level of respect even if we didn't understand it totally as we were just kids. But respect was given without question because of a uniform.

Sadly in a few places, kids are taught to disrespect people in uniforms. The police are likely treated the worst, but some calls referred to them as "pigs." That made me feel bad for them and I can understand how it would not make you happy to "Serve and to Protect." As EMS, we are treated much more civilly on most days but we too can be treated the same as the police on some calls. The days of not needing backup or a personal protection vest are long gone. The only solution is to respect everyone who deserves it especially in the first few encounters. If we keep getting disrespect when we provide our professionalism, the ability to nurture or to create a unique bond of trust is much more difficult to achieve. The calls when the patient smiles at you despite the fact they have a broken leg you know you're at the most appropriate level to help your patient.

Empathy is something we don't learn up front in life. We don't learn to deal with it in school or at least I never got that course. I would watch Sarah attend and she had a style that was different from my style of patient care but in the end, we had the same result. I would use humour and therapeutic touch and she would use an honest caring attitude. She had a voice that soothed most patients in pain and decreased their anxiety. We both felt others' pain or we perceived it enough to know the reasons why they needed our help. It was not a time to debate whether someone could be or might be a "drug seeker" or if they were not really that sick. We just treated the pain they claimed to have or sedated them with our wonderful medications and transported them with tender loving care (TLC) as well as provided them with the emotional and the compassionate care needed for the situation all at the same time.

All in all, we wanted our patients to feel they mattered. Even some of the worst situations required professionalism. We needed to ensure we were not the judge or the jury without all the facts. Our physician co-workers had figured that out much better than we had, but maybe it was because we were such a new profession. We had to grow but to grow as a profession we needed to spend the time required learning the lessons of life as well. Not all lessons are learned overnight, I had to remind myself over and over during my career.

We are often attracted to the people we are most like on many occasions. The attraction can be seen as affection but on a professional level it is much deeper. When we find the right working partner we actually become devoted to their safety and, their personal needs, and we display a friendly approach to each other at all times. If we had the wrong partner we would be challenging them on many parts of the call and the days would be much longer than they needed to be for the wrong reasons.

With the right partner, the time flies and before you know it on some days, the shift is over. On many calls, I would watch over my partners to ensure no harm ever came their way. If it did, I would stand in front of the harm and take the problem head on. A few times it cost me several stitches and sometimes a pair of glasses but it was the right thing to do. My belief was that you would or could not hit a lady. My partners Lisa and Sarah were ladies in all the right ways so I stood my ground to defend them at any cost. Even if I got a few looks from my partner I was okay as long as they knew I was their backup if needed.

What makes the right partner is the ability to have fun and do our difficult job at the same time. For almost every shift I went to work in a good mood, despite the bad nights or the bad sleep I'd had. I would not or could not be a jerk to anyone for any reason unless they were evil and then I would distance myself from them; that was my way of dealing with them. Many times, at work we would have so much fun we almost got in trouble a few times. Yes, we did play many jokes on people and we created some laughter from time to time with our backup crews or the nurses when we came in smiling from our crazy calls.

When you're dealing with life and death situations you need some level of detachment as well as a sense of humour at the right time to break the tension. As long as no one is being put down or made to feel bad, most things were appropriate. But we know certain medications that make you want to go to the bathroom to void can start the fizzing process that just won't quit when added to diet coke – we found out the hard way. But the funniest one was to turn on the emergency flashing lights, the siren on yelp as well as the heater on maximum in the back when they turned on the master power switch. We were just warming the unit up for them you could say.

We never got in trouble but we were brought to the supervisor's office a few times. In the end, we took our beating, went back to work and laughed all the way to Timmy's. One night I was so tired when we went into the ER for a STAT transfer out with a very sick patient I had to really push myself to stay awake and realize I was on a real call. The patient presented with a decreased level of consciousness (LOC) due to a multi-pharmacy and alcohol overdose with the intent to go to a better place. It was just another tragic day for a sad individual having a really bad day.

Over the years, I was fairly good but I only did the male catheters when needed and I would get one of the female nurses to do the female catheters for obvious reasons. It just made such a private procedure more comfortable for everyone. Several nurses had tried to get the catheter in and I said to them all right up front "I'm good with the male anatomy," as that was what I had and females were just different so they were not my specialty. But I will try just the same to get the catheter placed so we can get going. Well in a little bit I had a catheter draining from just the right magic opening with clear yellow urine. I had found the right spot and placed a special tube at the right opening at the right time. Everyone was smiling and cheering me on for they had tried multiple times. I looked at the nurses and said the line from Denzel Washington "Who's your Daddy?" from the movie "Remember the Titans" as a motivational speech. It was all in fun and the patient piped up and told us her dad's name very clearly and then passed out again. I almost died laughing as did the rest of the nurses in the room. Just a few minutes before they were going to intubate her as she was unresponsive, suddenly awoken and then in about ten seconds she had passed out again. My line had way more meaning than I was thinking in the early morning hours. That one hard laughing spell gave me a few extra hours of life.

The tour ended after our one final transfer. I was done and sleep was my next essential nourishment requirement. All in all, I could not have asked for better partners for so many reasons. We each had our strengths and our weaknesses. Overall, my partner was my safety net and I was theirs. Even on the easy calls they had our back. Some days when you're tired and almost exhausted any extra edge helping people is worthy.

Chapter 19: The Lost Soul

"The Only Way Out Alive"

The part that we could never predict is when we would do the bad calls were bad or which calls would or could affect us the most. There would be certain calls that would be physically and mentally exhausting in almost inhuman ways but we got through them unscathed. They were very taxing for our brain and tested our knowledge on so many levels. At the same time, the calls were all chronically increasing your rate of awareness and, your metabolic rates. You almost always would be on edge in order to do your ultimate best 24/7. Your brain and your body would constantly be receiving extra sensory input and your level of consciousness would also be just be more elevated while responding or performing the complete call. You just took the good calls with the bad calls and as a team you made them as successful as possible. Thankfully, someone was always looking out for us at so many levels. We were able to intervene as often as we could to prevent additional suffering and abort a terrible situation when it was meant to happen.

The rate of stressful calls would always be particular to your own service area. You would always have certain EMS services that would be more taxing to the staff than other services. We would also see certain staff that somehow missed the bad calls and some staff that got more than their fair share of the bad calls. The busiest services were great for experience but sometimes the bad calls also increased statistically just as the normal routine calls did as well.

On a normal service, the stressful calls were far apart and the practitioner would have time to recover in between the bad ones. The worst-case scenario was sadly displayed to many of the staff that knew Greg Turner as an example of the worst ending of a life of any EMS member. Greg was a very good seasoned paramedic who over a short period of time witnessed or was involved in many tragic calls. Sadly, he was not able to reach out, or to share his pain with people who could help him and to stabilize himself. The practitioners who worked with him or knew him will never forget that terrible day. There were many people who would have done anything for him but didn't get the chance. All we can do for the rest of time is to assume his caring and nurturing character and carry on his legacy to help others despite the situation and let him live in all of us.

The repeated stressful calls can push anyone of us too far towards our maximal coping limit. Every staff member had different limits due to their ability to learn or master some type of good coping mechanisms. Most are fortunate enough to be around the right staff to debrief, to unwind that was so helpful after the bad calls. When you had a bad call and you could talk about it with people that understood, it helped you lessen your pain enough to carry on because the next serious call was just around the corner. We often could always provide each other with extra support when needed and it really lessened the accumulation of harmful stress. Just knowing you could go out after a bad or stressful shift with a good friend and share your stories over a coffee or beverage was a very beneficial way to vent the stress. It was one step forward thus keeping you a little further away from greater personal harm. To the ones that went home and drank alcohol to lessen the pain they only delayed the resolution or healing of the real pain.

The one thing the repeated or busy calls would or could do to anyone of us was: it could bring you closer to the edge, either to being really good in your job or being over the edge of being therapeutic or helpful in any real emergency. The push to make you better and better as a practitioner was almost always healthy but not over time. The one thing that could affect us all was the calls that would not go away. Looking back, we all had our own bad calls that took over our soul from time to time. We would have calls that took our soul and broke it to little pieces. They were the ones that we needed help to get over. Most times it was our co-workers helping to reach out to help us, but the real support came from the emergency staff that received some of the worst of our patients. They were our real support.

When we walked into our local ER and I could see one of my nursing friends such as Lynn, Joanne, Jacqueline, Tana, Rebecca, Mandy, Bondy, Melinda, Shelby, Erika, Randie-Lynn, or almost any of our current emergency physicians, we had hope every time of helping the sick and injured. We also had many other team members that were ready to battle any situation with us with no questions, but too many to name. There are so many more others involved from the admitting staff, the radiology staff, the laboratory staff, that I can't name them all but just know you all matter. You're all part of the reason we are successful with in-patient care and with our overall career outcomes. Many of our favourites would give us strength and endurance to keep going after the bad calls. After some of my bad days I would go and find Leanne and got a hug. After I had a really bad day I would stop and cry on her shoulder and she held me up despite me being more than twice her size. To me people that cared gave me life. Everyone needed a guardian angel.

The calls that broke me or made me different over time were the broken kids and the wrongful deaths of others. We often were called to assist with the senseless deaths as the most stressful calls. The repeated injuries from abuse, physical assault and the new realization of the elder abuse cases are troublesome for all rescuers.

At the end of the day we really need to realize we are just part of the essential emergency responders that have been selected to help our patient's outcomes after any illness or injury. Over the years, I was always a little more aggressive in the management of people who needed our support more than the others. This would almost always be the kids, the elderly or the special population groups such as the handicapped or mentally and psychically challenged. When people needed someone to help them or someone at their side, it was our battle. We proudly accepted the challenge.

Not everyone we were called to assist actually wanted our help. I realized that If you were an adult with no drugs or alcohol on board and you hated your life and wanted to die it was an option. I would often feel bad for you but you can refuse our care if you met the right criteria. Your life is yours and if you're alert and oriented x 4 spheres and you don't want help, we can't fix you. We can ask the police to help us and try to get the patient brought in under the Mental Health Act, but sometimes the system is not going to help us to help you get better.

Some people can be just miserable and unhappy with life in general. Sometimes we can't help everyone in need and the more we try the worse the situation escalates to the point we could be at risk of harm. Every time I run across someone that is really nasty and not nice to any of us my patience is pushed. I'm so thankful to see the nice people on the next call. They soon would cancel out the evil that people have inside them waiting to pounce on the nice people in this world. It's easy to be nice to good people.

We often will come across the people in this world that have come to the end of their rope and are almost the lost souls of this world. The only way to reach them from our perspective is to show them we actually care about everyone the same. Often people might have seen unmeasurable tragedy before our meeting. Many have lost loved ones, lost their kids, been divorced, or may have had a big financial loss which brings them to feel they have no other options but death.

Sometimes this hopelessness will come from a person after they have had a significant loss of a loved one that can be devastating.

We often see couples that have been married for many years and when they lose their significant partner they are also lost or beyond broken. The one call I remember that breaks my heart was after we coded a loved one we ended up calling the code on scene and it broke the patient's spouse's heart. It was a day we all lost something but gained something else. We all got to see the most human side of life and to also witness unconditional love.

The poor lady just wanted to say goodbye her way. She asked me and I said sure. Then she simply crawled in beside him and just held him tight and cried. All we could do was to support her for as long as she needed to say her goodbye. Sometimes the best healing comes from the family being able to share their love and affection even after their partner has passed away. The internal healing will come from the ones they have loved the most for a lifetime and that's part of the healing process that is needed after the loss of a loved one. So please, never assume after we call a cardiac arrest that our job is done. Some days that's when the real work starts in our world. Every nurse or EMS staff member who has seen multiple cardiac arrests will have seen this as part of loss and the most important part of the grieving process. How we handle the initial grieving period makes many able to let go of such a valued part of their life.

The worst I've seen is a parent that just lost a child in a traumatic case. The worst situation is often when only one person or one family member survives and the rest are killed. Even if it was an accident, their life is going to be greatly affected. Just know that we can't or won't be able to fix everything. Some days we are limited in our ability to fix very much at all. People need time to grieve and this is something we can help with initially but sadly not in a timely or for a long period of time. It's good to get the right people to support the survivors as soon as possible, if at all possible to come and relieve us as soon as possible (ASAP). Then the pain of the loss can have a better outcome for the survivor in time to come. The loss of a child often makes parents lives changed for the rest of their lives.

Sometimes if we can only give our patients some hope, or we showed them that we cared, it's a good start. If we at least show them we care they were will have someone on their side in a time of crisis. One person on your side in this big bad world on your side is what some people need for a reason to live. Some days we are that one person that will care and that simple gesture shows that they have something to live for. Then they will know they matter. It's a start and that is more then we can hope for in many cases.

When we arrived on scene and find the patient in a confused state and disorientated to the normal events around them, we have a good reason to transport them, despite them not wanting our help. I would commonly not give anyone an option about coming with us. The odd time it's a battle to get them to seek help but on average it is just another routine sick person call. Most times it is easy, as we just need to convince them to go to the right hospital for an assessment and some much-needed medical treatment. After all, once we are called and have arrived on scene it's easy enough to convince them after all someone must have called us. We are more than ready and willing to get them to a local ER for essential help in most cases.

It is often easy to find a reason to transport them if you actually wanted to get them out of an unhealthy environment from time to time. It's also easy to find a reason *not* to transport them if you really looked hard but I was never in favour of cancellations in almost all circumstances, unless the call was really bogus or not justified at all. We would often get called for trivial events and sometimes it is hard to even understand why the dispatcher even put the call through. But after all they were doing their job and that was the way it was. Just know our dispatchers are not the real gatekeepers against the abuse of EMS or to the hospitals. They do stop some of the silliest calls before we get dispatched from time to time.

If you really have someone who needs to be transported we do our best to ensure they go to the hospital. I can count on one hand the cases where EMS made a really bad judgement call. Sadly, we transported to a few rural and urban emergency rooms where the nurses were not very happy to ever see us and we would get the "Why would you bring them to us?" speech. All too often a few nurses were very rude at one hospital we often would transport to. I would do my utmost best to avoid any hospital that was reluctant to care about people in need. It was simply an ethical and moral problem for me. When we had a reason to be dispatched, it was often easier to take the patient to the local ER and let the hospital decide if it was trivial or not. All we needed to do was simply show we were concerned about them or explain that they need much more help than we could provide. Even after being rude or thankless to us they both often would turn to the patients and become nice again to our sick or injured patient. That was what really mattered in the end.

Many times, we found that our sick patients had altered vital signs such as low oxygen levels, or the blood sugars too low or too high or that something was wrong with their clinical or physical assessment. Every once in awhile, the outcome was bad despite the ability of the crew to get them transported for help. Sometimes their circumstances were not good no matter what we did, or their physical health was terrible or their diagnosis was a terminal event regardless of our helpful approach. All we could do was show we cared and that someone actually wanted to help them. Destiny and fate would look after the rest. Sadly, time was not always long for our sickest patients.

On one of the normal days Sarah would always keep me looking ahead and positive even when I was having a hard day walking or standing straight and tall. I found that for some reason I was thinking more and more about the lost souls in our world. I wondered why we had so many homeless or too many people living in poverty while others were wasteful and extravagant. It just made no sense to me that in the modern world we could not fix the most broken areas of our cities. One night on a transfer I was looking out of the window and as we travelled down the four-lane highway I could see lights in the middle of nowhere.

I wondered how we could have streetlights from our biggest city all the way to the Edmonton International Airport (EIA) on both sides of the Queen Elizabeth II Highway all while some of our seniors were starving or did not have enough money for their required prescription medications. Then when I started adding up the cost of just this one huge extra cost to taxpayers it made me sad. It would be about twenty to twenty-five kilometers of streetlights on both sides of the highway and then you had to power them year-round. "Why would we spend that type of money which was in the many millions, yet neglect our elderly?" was my simple but unanswered question left in my mind to wonder. Or perhaps we cut the educational funding to many schools or secondary educational institutions, just so people wouldn't need to use their headlights on a well-travelled highway, when darkness is not ever an issue any ways – it's purely a waste of energy and resources.

Ironically, when cars lose control on the Queen Elizabeth II Highway they frequently hit the light stands. Then the poles are knocked over, which I'm guessing would cost thousands per pole; the upkeep and power needed would run a small rural farm, I'm sure. Our society needs to stop and refocus on the real needs of our people and not the dream world.

Then the simple fact we moved the STARS base to the Edmonton International Airport (EIA) due to political and financial reasons affected more people than they bargained for I'm sure. It cost our STARS helicopter more to do mandatory training and I'm sure that was never even considered. Someone told me it was a $50 fee for take-off or for a landing fee and in a day of training that would add up to a considerable increased overall cost very quickly. Thankfully the surrounding airports had no service fees or charges so we got to see them training in Wetaskiwin for free which was a win-win for the local residents that admire watching the helicopters land and to takeoff on frequent training maneuvers. Many days the golden retrievers and I simply stopped our outside adventure to admire their flying skills.

I think the Edmonton Municipal Airport was doomed for years in our province but, as in many things, we change but not always for the right reasons. Some people would get richer by closing the airport and others such as very sick patients would have to survive longer ground transport during an EMS transport ride, the cost of which was just added to the cost of progress. We had a good system for all air ambulance operations and then one day the system was made more complicated and the cost was doubled, but that didn't matter! Change was part of what we needed to function in a changing society. Not all changes are for the right reasons but that's not our concern – for we just have to accept the change and pay our taxes, despite the waste or the broken systems it creates.

On the upside, the STARS base was closer to the people in my home EMS area so our rotary aircraft back up was much closer. As in everything there is always good in something, but only from one person's perspective. If you lived on the north side of Edmonton the STARS flying time was longer so all in all everything had circumstances that were both bad and good. It is funny that as you get older or mature you would see things that for years you simply took for granted. Sarah would see the world from a completely different perspective than I would have, but I'm from a different era in the time continuum so it' was not something that I can or would ever change. Even if it made me concerned, it was not something I would be able to change in my remaining life span.

One day I was talking to Sarah while we were waiting for a call and nothing was happening in our base all day long, which was very rare. The radio messages and the calls all around us were all bad and the events around us on the CAD were also all bad. Multiple serious calls and bad accidents were happening everywhere and we were smiling, sitting doing nothing. I said to Sarah, "This world is simply going straight to hell my friend." We were seeing the bad stuff daily and it seemed the abuse of drugs and domestic abuse calls were on the rise for every service as well. Sarah smiled at me and then punched me lightly in the shoulder. She said, "Don't lose faith, my friend, especially on our bad days."

The good days happen for a specific reason, just as the bad days have a unique reason as well. We needed the bad days to better appreciate the good days even more. I thought about it and she was right. I was not looking forward with my head up or my vision was not clear from the fog of badness in the world around us. Sometimes life can do that to us, even if we don't even realize it's happening. I just needed to look further out of my regular visual fields to see the good as well as the bad events.

Many days I just about gave up on society and the caring about the general public. Maybe I was just not seeing the good side of life for I lacked my inner spirit's good or positive voice. My partners could see that in seconds. The tone of my voice and my posture said everything even without hearing the words. Sometimes we needed our partners to pick us up and point us in the right direction. It's easy to get lost and have no vision if you hold your head too far down and lose your faith in humanity. It seems to happen to me more often these days than in my past years. I wish I understood the why but I did not.

Thinking about our job, I realized our service had thrived on other problems. We would never be without a job. Our call volume was on the rise as we were creating a world that needed us more and more due to the unhealthy life styles of many of our patients. People were doing unhealthy activities or simply making deadly life choices on daily occurrences. Many of the people doing the more potent drugs all had a reason to need a medication high or a boost to bring them out of a deep dark place. We would then see the death rates triple and the cost to our healthcare system increase or possibly double due to the higher demands because of the side effects of such toxic abuse of drugs but we simply have no solutions.

We are now charged with finding a solution for other people's drug problems in record numbers and even if it was only Narcan® it was something that I noticed. In the end, the senseless high was needed and people would risk anything to get the boost from a bad place. This made no logical sense to me after seeing people fighting to live and dying despite wanting to live; it was not fair. Life was never fair to certain people suffering but then that was and is always part of life. Sadly, many had everything to live for but died just for that one good high that took their life in seconds. The only grace would be to know that they had no pain in the end. The only scary part would be when the sympathetic system tripled its side effect to fight or flight. It kicked in to prevent death, for a mere second that part would have been pure hell, and then it was over.

Sarah and I talked for hours. When we both came to the conclusion that to heal we needed to get rid of the inner bitterness, throw away the rage or the bad emotions, and we needed to forget about personal slander that people often gave us as it brings us all down. We needed to be better than that and we had to fight the good fight; and regardless of the outcome we had to live for the good things. I honestly had lost some hope but after thinking about the good versus the bad outcome that was always around us we had many more good things than we actually realized. It's easy to get tunnel vision in life, in living and for our future.

To win or lose our battle in our lifetime of helping people, we needed to fight the good fight and just do our job. Regardless of the outcome, we had to carry on and we needed to start counting our wins more often than just our loses. It was the only way to help make us see the best in the world around us. Somehow the good needed to be sought out and brought out of the hiding spots. I was so thankful to be with a partner that actually cared about people more than life itself, for she always knew my innermost feelings and had my back 24/7. The odds of me finding her as a partner and as a best friend was most likely about one in a billion.

Sometimes we are pushed to our personal limits for a good reason. We need to stretch our abilities to help the people in the greatest need for the obvious reason. We would be called to calls that are true-life emergencies. The priority would be surrounding the effort of the patient's breathing or perhaps the respiration was ineffective and that was a starting point in our care. Often the heart was taking a partial holiday. It could be a slow or fast heart rate as it was being blocked out or stimulated either chemically or by the structural defects within the heart.

Then we would try to deal with the perfusion issues at lightning speed that we assessed upon our arrival. We would often walk into hell some days and we never complained, we just went to work and we made the best out of a bad patient presentation. One day I would do one set of skills and the next day I would do something else. We always had it worked out before we arrived unless the situation dictated a quick change. The biggest determination would be the level of consciousness as a deciding factor on stable, unstable or in a worst case a respiratory cardiac arrest.

On many calls, we would sense a feeling of fight or flight and some days it was a feeling of doom right away. We often knew when people had simply given up and the soul was long gone. We could only do our best and the rest was up to someone else. We were just specially trained personnel and in the right place at the right time, we were successful. At the wrong place in time surrounded with bad events the decisions were already final. All we needed was some hope and we were off to the races to save a life.

Sometimes the evil world brings us down but a good person or a positive message would lift us back up. We could go from one call where we would laugh and laugh at certain parts of the call when it was appropriate. We actually got several of our patients laughing so hard they would almost pass out. But we could and we would bring them back. It was all the same charge. The only thing that would and did break our spirit was the evil, or repeated negative events. Good and evil are part of the world we live in and everyone knows that we must see both in our line of work. On the worst calls we would see the hell people live in such as, the pain they received from the beatings or the severe pain from being stabbed or from being shot. For the most part, they were the innocent ones in most cases.

Every once in awhile, karma would pay back evil with evil but we were not the judges – we just tried our best to keep the good and the bad patients alive. We were rewarded for both situations. In the best of the times the good events would help bury the bad events and that was soothing to many of us. I wouldn't wish bad times on anyone but when another bad person takes out drug dealers, the abusers of others I didn't lose any sleep. Once and awhile I would try to think of a time when the drug dealer was a kid and wonder why they made the choices they made. The system makes evil multiply just as good also spreads love and caring throughout the world. Just know that some good comes from bad things and that bad can come from some good.

The troubles we see in the healthcare world and in the real world can eat at our soul even in small pieces from time to time. I realized in the end of my career I had to get out intact. I had to quit on a good note. I knew the world would not heal overnight. I said this to

Sarah and her comeback was from something she was reading on her iPad. It was simple: "Just know people won't remember what we say. People won't remember what we do for them. But people will remember how we made them feel." That was what had to matter on a bad day. That was what mattered to most people we touched or helped. That good feelings we get also raises us back up on a bad day even more. On my worst days, I had to know we had made a difference. I had to know we often made the right decisions, even if sometimes we lost our way more than what people ever would see from the outside looking in.

My only way out from a bad day was with the help of my partner. Sarah had saved me just as I had saved her. We smiled and looked into each other's hearts and I said thank you and just like that our tones went off. "Nine-Echo" which is a cardiac arrest at a local restaurant. Today we would not get off on time. Today we would be pushed to the limits, but we both knew that as we hit the streets at high speed with our emergency lights flashing and our siren screaming away. We had a cardiac arrest waiting for our small bag or handful of miracles. We would try and abort a bad outcome with our skills, our combined wisdom and our team effort we would try our best to bring this person back alive.

If by a small miracle, we could help save one more soul we would make it happen. We had everything to win and one more soul to lose. As we were a block away, Medic-Three Tim and Tina just came around the next intersection and were coming in hot and fast right at us. Today our backup was coming even before being dispatched. Today we had the right teams and today we would save a life. I just knew it. We could both feel it already. I reached over and gave Sarah a high five and said, "Let's kick some butt, my lady." I just thought to myself: "Please don't be a kid." Anything but a kid I could handle today or at least I would get through it without one more prematurely lost soul to worry about. Then my mind went to the list of differential diagnosis and then we were hitting the brakes hard.

Time was against us but also on our side today. No matter what we walked into we were a team and that was what really mattered at the end of the day.

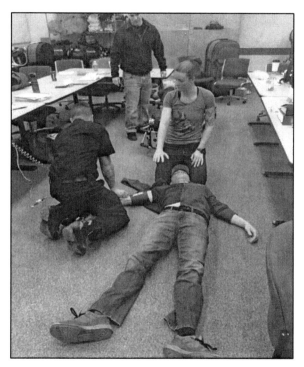

"With the Right Team We Win Every time despite the Outcomes"

Chapter 20: The Final Battle for a Life

"Time to Walk Away"

I would say the biggest challenge we have in our EMS and medical careers is to save lives. When people had gone into cardiac arrest or if they'd arrested in front of us that was the greatest challenge. It was always shocking to be talking to someone and suddenly they were pulseless, apneic and just gone. It was then up to us to figure out the many causes of the respiratory or cardiac arrest and try our best to get them back in a timely fashion. Every second matters and every minute counted against us if we had no real signs of life. When we got them back we would be in heaven ourselves for a few seconds. That one pure feeling meant something special to all of us, it was a special feeling you can't ever forget.

We can all look back and declare the wins from our many calls; even if they are only short-lived wins they still count. If we found someone in cardiac arrest and we got them to the hospital with a pulse it was a win. The thirty-day discharge window wasn't as promising but that was not our immediate concern. We could only do our best for as long as we had patient contact. The next part was up to the excellent care in the ER by the nurses, the doctors, and the lab and X-ray staff. In all, we would try to decide what was the biggest threat to life and those factors would be challenged. It was rare but sometimes people would not live after getting them back stable and talking, but it did happen. We would get them back and think we had saved them but a secondary threat would come along and we would lose. Those hurt us more than people could ever see. We always wanted to do our best and if we lost someone even if they were elderly they were still someone's family.

Many times, we would get the patients back on the scene or in the ER and then it was someone else's job to maintain life signs in at least a semi-stable condition. As soon as they could be sent out to a receiving hospital they would be packaged and sent out by STARS or by a ground unit with the most appropriate level of care. In Alberta, it just depended on where you lived as to which mode of transport worked best. We were most fortunate that the receiving hospitals were almost always more than accommodating – if they could make us a bed they would, and then it was up to the transport crews to keep the patient stable. Many transports were uneventful once they were stabilized but sometimes the transports were complete disasters. Despite trying to be prepared, things could always go wrong. I would never realize until after patient care was transferred to the waiting critical care teams that bad luck was dead ahead.

After arrival at the city ERs or the ICUs, the real battle for life started. The organ dysfunctions, the multiple system failures and the repeated efforts of our patients to die would start. In the end, if our survivors were meant to live it would happen. Some days we were just meant to lose some of our battles to save a life despite our best efforts. I have seen many calls go very well but every once in awhile, suddenly the patient deteriorates and our second chance to bring them back is a futile effort. We never knew when and where some of our patients would run out of time and just like that they would be lost, despite our efforts to revive them.

On one transport Sarah was attending and I was just listening to the talk from the back of the unit. Sarah was so genuine and her caring nature was always up front. This made me think about all the other staff we worked with and I realized we are not all the same. The one thing that some people take for granted is that we all must care. Well despite the idea, it's not always the case. I had seen multiple staff members get upset as soon as the tones go off – did they think they were just hired to fill in a shift vacancy? We always worked as a team. Our calls and transports were something we looked forward to, they made the days so much more fulfilling.

Then I wondered why some of the other crews never wanted to go on the calls or seemed to be inconvenienced when they were toned out. I was trying to decide if it was burnout, lack of caring or simply a lack of motivation in life itself. When you were with the right partner responding to emergency calls or doing the transfers it was a challenge and always an expected event. We needed to always be genuine and caring while trying to be positive despite the mixed-up world around us. It was the hardest when we were called to the worst of the worst and we kept seeing the bad parts of life more than we could see the winning parts so we were a little jaded in our outlook in life, I'm sure. I would see this happen from time to time after we had a busy night and not enough sleep. We all get tired. But at the end of the day we still must care for everyone at the same level.

Our second day shift was a busy morning with three calls back to back for mostly minor events but they still took time. We stopped at Timmy's and always got our coffees to go in case we ended up leaving in a hurry. Sarah was responding to some work-related emails and I was just relaxing. I was sitting watching the people come and go. It made me wonder what most people would do if they could do anything they wanted to in the world. We would see nice people coming for coffee and it looked like it was a routine they did every day as their order was already in the staff member's head and they were ringing in the order as they walked towards the till. They called the person by name and they were smiling at each other so it was a win-win for all parties. It would make the day just a little more rewarding in such a low-paying position.

Then out of the blue someone who was just cranky would come and be abusive to the staff despite the opening smile. I guess not every person comes to get a coffee to be sociable. Some have a control issue or enjoy causing others harm, as they seem to take joy in being unpleasant to the staff that are trying to do their best. I felt sorry for the staff because if the same person were nasty to me I would ensure they had better medications pushed into their medication port to control some of their anger management issues. We had medications that could make the worst of the worst as quiet as a sleeping cat. Timmy's staff had to smile and take it, which seemed so unfair. It was like watching a bully-training video from a bystander's perspective.

Only once did I need to step forward. I was inline when a bully was very nasty to a young teller and after a bit of him getting worse and worse I intervened. I asked the cashier if this nasty person came here all the time and he spun around – I was daring him to take a poke at me. I was not about to let him be nasty and rude to a teenage girl trying to make some money at a part-time job. He walked away and grunted some swear words at me and she smiled and thanked me. I smiled back and I said, "You're more than welcome." I bet he thought twice about being rude to anyone for a bit. Thankfully he decided that to battle me was a losing idea and walked away or we would have had some explaining to do when I called 911 for someone who fell and slipped in front of me. It would have been a nasty quick fall I was sure.

We had just got back in the unit and were driving back to the base when we were called to respond to a shooting. It was an accidental shooting and tragically a child has been shot. The RCMP was already responding so we just followed them out of town to back them up as fast as possible. Sarah was driving and I was on the phone to the dispatch centre. STARS were on a mission and our backup was coming from a greater distance but they were still coming. Today we would be alone with the RCMP officers as well as the volunteer Fire Department that was to be dispatched; however, they were also fighting a fire so they were running short of staff. They would still free up someone anyway. Today the systems were all being taxed with the current call volumes. We were about two minutes from being on scene and we were updated by dispatch that the scene was secure. The first police were on scene. Then they updated us to hurry. We could not possibly go faster but we were trying.

As we pulled into the farmyard we saw the police, the county peace officers and a sheriff's vehicle all around the driveway as we entered the scene. We parked as close as we could to the group of people gathered. I said to Sarah as we pulled up "I hate kid calls." Sarah grabbed my hand and said to me with pure determination "We've got this, my friend," but we already knew it was going to be a bad one. I jumped out and grabbed our trauma kit and Sarah grabbed the LP-15 cardiac monitor. We approached to see a young child covered in blood all over her right chest. She looked about seven or eight years old as we walked up to her. The dad was distraught and the police were intervening with him as best possible. One police officer said to us both it was an accidental shooting. She was hit once in the chest with a 22-calibre bullet. It was such a nasty injury and the calibre smaller than most shootings, but to a small kid it was very significant. With one look, we knew it was very bad. Despite only being a small entrance hole, the injury inside was terrible and most likely it would do a devastating amount of damage. Most likely the bullet broke up after it hit a rib and then it would do triple the internal damage. It was the mushrooming effect of a smaller calibre bullet but it was never meant to hit this kid.

We quickly applied a bulky dressing over the injury to slow the blood loss. One of the first officers had already applied a field dressing from his first aid kit but it had soaked right through in seconds. We found her alive and she was gasping for air. She was fighting for every breath. She was still trying to talk to us as well but her words were incomprehensible. Her colour was a terrible grey and she was soaked in sweat already. Her heart was fighting to beat as long as possible. We log rolled her and ensured there was not bad bleeding from an exit on her back. We placed her on a long spine board that one of the officers had brought from the unit. My brain was working at lightning speed. We needed an OR. We don't have access to one. We needed blood. We had none. We needed a chest tube. We didn't have one. We needed STARS and they were not coming. We needed a miracle and we needed it right now.

I said to Sarah, "Let's move to the unit and make a run for the ER. If we stay on scene she dies." She nodded her head but never said a word. She was thinking. Sarah was trying to come up with the only chance this girl would get to live I just knew it. As Sarah was coming up with the only plan that would work I let her work on it as I was worried about the more immediate stuff. I was getting my mind ready for our attack in the unit. We would do nothing at all on scene as we would just be wasting precious seconds and lifesaving minutes. Today it was real-life scoop and run and then drives as fast as we could possibly go. We had an eighteen to twenty-minute transport time at normal speed but at high speed we could make it in fourteen – or fifteen minutes and that was driving wide open. It was just too far and we were running out of time. She had no more blood to lose. She looked so pale, but by some miracle she was still fighting to live. She was so small but she had more fight in her. She was living despite the real fact she had nothing left to fight with. But she would not quit.

Then Sarah said in a matter of factual way, "Let's get the blood to meet us." We also needed the ER doctor. "Let's get an ER doctor to come to us with the blood." I said, "Let's try." I looked at the senior officer. "Get a member to go to the local ER, grab the blood, a doctor with chest tubes and meet us on the highway." We will meet in the middle. We have nothing to lose and a little life to gain. Sarah took my iPhone and speed-dialled the local ER, as her phone was not in reach. She spoke to the charge nurse and arranged a miracle in the making.

The request was done in seconds. At the same time, I was trying to help her breathe with a BVM as we were loading her into the unit. Every bit of help was being made possible. We had an officer at every corner of the stretcher taking her safely to the unit. Ben the senior member was holding the dressing as tightly as possible to slow the external blood loss from the right chest injury. I asked for a driver and I also asked for a member to help in the back and it was arranged. I reached over and stuck a big needle in her small right chest to decompress the rapidly accumulating pneumothorax that I would be making worse with the BVM. That was one of the consequences of our best intentions on a bad day.

I would be giving her the much-needed oxygen but the lacerated torn lung would be weeping and running blood in the path of the broken projectile. It helped a little bit to enable her to breathe but it was not enough. This little angel never even cried when I stuck the needle in her but her eyes were actually looking at us and pleading for life. I was trying with everything I could to give her more life. We needed a surgeon, we needed the blood as well as the chest tube.

We were off of the scene in less than two minutes with some simple instructions to our commandeered driver. Go really easy on the corners and 'giver' on the straight roads. We may have already lost this battle, but we were going to give this little lady every possible chance. There was just too much bleeding and the blood loss was just too much. It was just too much internal lung and tissue damage. There was not one person against us that day on scene or on the roads. Nothing would or could have stopped us. We would try to defeat every known obstacle before it even came up.

After we left the scene I was working on her airway. I was giving her high flow oxygen and setting up to intubate her while assisting her breathing a little with the BVM. She kept coughing up blood on me but I never even noticed. Sarah had an IV in right away and was running it wide open. Next, we both applied parts of the monitor and our commandeered officer was pressure infusing the IV solution with his hands of steel. Our driver was calling off the corners and we were moving as fast as we could travel. We had several RCMP vehicles in front of us and an extra one behind us. Other members would deal with the scene and someone would be bringing the dad as soon as possible but that was not our problem or priority right now. His hell would not be over for days to come but at least we gave him some hope. It was all anyone could ever expect.

I could hear the officer's radio with our movements being called off and the unit that was meeting us talking back and forth with one of the police cars. They had kept the police channel open for us and no one was able to interfere with our mission. As we approached the highways and any major intersection, the first police vehicle in the lead stopped all opposing traffic and we didn't stop or slow down. Then after we went through the intersection he would take over being the trailing vehicle and our rear escort moved ahead to cover our front. They had the advantage of reaching much higher speeds than we could as we were such a heavy vehicle and unable to exceed our governed speed of 140 km/hr. They were running interference down the highway as well and no one was in our way.

In no time, they had the blood and, doctor and in several minutes, they were coming from the local ER right to us at high speed. They would be moving like a jet towards us with an expert driver making time seem to slow down. Our closing speed would have been over 300 km/h. It was faster than any helicopter and it was on the open roads with nothing to obstruct our meeting. The miracle was coming to us and we were transporting the precious angel right to the only place in time that mattered to any of us.

We planned a meeting point that was easy and a middle point for all of us. They had one fire rescue truck that was setting up a place to meet. When we met, they would jump in and declare battle the military way. We would fight this injury on the side of the road. It would be our last stand. If we could save this little lady it would be done on our terms. If it were at all possible we would win despite the losing hand we'd been dealt that terrible day. Losing was never an option once we got going. The momentum that was made left only one option – we had to win. The win was our only option.

I needed to secure an airway but I had her clenching on my fingers still. I then gave her a little bit of medication but just enough to get her to let me intubate her. It was all I needed as she was in such bad state of shock it was hardly needed at all. The BP was maybe 40 systolic with a heart rate of 160 bpm. The oxygen saturations were not registering which was making me extra scared. Sarah was starting another IV and was setting up the blood tubing with a normal saline bag to flush the line wide open. All we needed was the blood.

My heart started to race and Sarah looked at me and said, "It's going to be okay. We will win this one." I had no idea how she knew it but her heart and soul knew we were to win. My heart immediately started to slow down again. My guardian angel was on my side even if I could not see her, I felt her at my side. Sarah was the only one in the world who would know the pure feelings I would be having right then. I was terrified we would lose despite the effort. Sarah was so positive we were going to win. I knew the rules of being the leader and still it was hard to keep control of the big picture.

The rules were simply that "Every good leader even in a losing battle must always show emotional stability to overcome all obstacles." It was easy in theory but some days the challenges are overwhelming. It was then that the other team members brought you back. Today Sarah was the one bringing me back. Together we had the ability to control the scene, the patient care and to make our transport decisions even better. It was the team spirit that saved us from pending disasters.

I contacted the ER and they were getting ready for us. They were also getting us more blood ready. They would also know that we were doing everything possible en route to try and save this one at any and all cost. We would not quit or let the angel of death take this one. This one child was sacred despite the fact we had never seen her in our whole life. Losing this battle was not an option. Well at least not without the biggest battle for a human life that was ever waged.

We would all work as a team of one and declare a final heroic battle that would come after such an innocent but deadly mistake from a loved one. I could not imagine how the dad must have felt after making such a tragic mistake. We were approaching the meeting point, and the highway was blocked off and we had a police car coming right at us at the speed of a small jet. We just needed a little help and it was in sight. We needed help but more than that we needed a miracle. That miracle was in sight. We just needed a few more seconds and it would be upon us.

I was trying to get another blood pressure (BP) reading. I could get a pulse but the BP was too low to even auscultate anymore. Her colour was so pale she was ghostly white now – it was scary. Her CO_2 was registering fifteen which means she was going to go into cardiac arrest without the blood. We had two IVs wide open and still no BP. We pulled into the meeting point and our back doors were flung open. In jumped one of our favourite ER nurses, an emergency room physician who was a gifted surgeon, as well as a family physician and also the emergency resident. They were the miracle we needed. Today we needed more help than imaginable and it was brought to us in the fastest way possible. Spock would have been proud of our actions! Even if he would not show any emotion, his heart would be smiling.

Our ER doctor was assessing, helping to try and stabilize the patient as soon as he had arrived. We had an update that STARS would be coming and would meet ASAP after their current flight at our local hospital ER. In no time, a chest tube was being inserted in the right side of the chest. The resident also put a chest tube in the opposite side and the breathing immediately got a little better. The nurse was working with Sarah and the blood was running in as fast as it would go. In no time at all the chest tubes were in and draining frankly large amounts of blood from the right chest, which was bad but expected.

We at least could ventilate a little better and slowly our oxygen levels were rising but we needed some hemoglobin (Hgb) for that. It was starting to run in as fast as possible. In no time, we had her starting to look alive again.

The doctor asked us to give TXA (Tranexamic acid) and we gave half the adult dose which was 500 mg and it was started right away over ten minutes. The resident surprised me even more as he was putting in a central line at the same time. Unknown to any of us he was training to be an emergency room physician and his skills were being put to the test. In less than five minutes we had started the convoy towards the local ER and with every single breath and every single heartbeat, life was being restored and preserved. We had made the transport the fastest possible trip in our history. No time was wasted at any point of the call. We just needed a little more time out of this broken angel and we would win. Over the last several minutes the odds were coming into our favour. This little lady was a fighter. It was like we were playing the world championship game and we had pulled our goalie in hopes of hitting the other's goal post with as much force as possible. We were taking the winning goal over the rest of the team and nothing at all would stop us.

We still could not get a measurable BP until we were almost at the local ER but the CO_2 was twenty-four now and the SpO_2 was registering at 90% which was better. It was not great but it was a start. Anything was better than what we had before the surgical interventions and the lifesaving blood. We were almost to the hospital when STARS made a low-level pass right past our racing convoy at a very low level. The ex-military pilot was just showing us his moral support in the only way he knew how. It was deeply appreciated. As we pulled into the local ER the crew and the ER staff swarmed us and they rapidly took over the life saving interventions. Rapidly the little lady was on the aircraft's stretcher, loaded in the running and waiting aircraft and they were off the ground in record time. They turned in the right direction using the tail winds to increase their speed and they were headed to the awaiting pediatric trauma team. There was nothing more we could do our job was done even if we ended up losing in the end we did more than our best to try and save a life.

Today we made a life come back from the wrong side of heaven. We pulled her back despite the horrific injury. I went back to our unit and took one look at the floor. It was literally soaked in bright red blood everywhere. There was garbage everywhere. We had completely torn our kits apart and had used everything possible to save a life. I had not seen so much blood loss from anyone. Our stretcher was saturated in blood. I then started to cry. I had just reached my limits. I had nothing left inside me to give. I just sat down and cried, leaning against the unit.

That is where they found me. My friends came and they found me broken and lost. They got down to my level, held me and we cried together. When it was over and I could see again I finally realized there was my friend Ben the police officer, one of the ER nurses, and my best friend who was the ER doctor on call. But the one that counted the most was my partner Sarah who was holding me the hardest. They took me to a private room and showed me I mattered. I said I had to go and clean my unit but I could not look at them, as I was so embarrassed until Ben grabbed my shoulders and said; "You have nothing to be embarrassed about. You have saved thousands and thousands." He looked at me as a friend. Ben said plainly, "We are your family too. What happens with us stays with us. Nobody can or should be ashamed about caring too much." We all needed each other today and in the end, we were only a team of one. I looked at Sarah and she looked at me. We were both still covered in so much, now dried blood but the blood was who we were. It was part of us. We earned it. We traded it for a life. We had given everything we had for one life.

It was just today I needed them as I had nothing left to give. They said it was being looked after. I was taken off shift and my workday was over. We all sat in a small room and slowly we started to share our stories about today. We shared our wins and we also shared some of our losses from the past. In the end, it was only about today. It was only about what we had just achieved. Soon it came around to the present call. The doctor was now in charge. He looked at us and said, "No matter what happens, she was given hope when hope was all but lost." There were no more miracles today to give out. We had used them all. She's still fighting for her life and they don't know yet but, regardless, we gave her time and with time she has hope. Sometimes that is all we can give people. Sarah held my hand and one of the nurses held the other one. I was surrounded by my friends. I apologized for breaking down. I don't know why but when I saw my unit soaked in blood I thought we had lost her despite the fact we tried so hard. I had never in my life seen so much blood cover everything. There was no way possible she could live with losing that much lifesaving blood. It was not possible.

They stopped me and said, "You are more than special, you are just too caring, my friend, and that's what makes us all human." Then we hugged each other even more. I started crying again but it was from the overwhelming love of my most loyal friends. You can't do this job and not be affected. It had built up to this after all these years. The breaking point to me was all that kid's blood. Before this call was done, we had given her enough IV fluid as well as blood to replace her blood volume about five times over in a very short order. Everything that came out of her was still good blood diluted in saline but it just came out of her in many buckets full and then simply ended up on the floor of the unit.

Slowly we had more police officers join into our group and a few more hospital staff. Then victim services asked to bring the family in. I was not sure if I could but sure enough I had to do this last part. It was my job. That was when I really started to cry but in a good way. In walked the parents and the same young girl I had stopped and helped that was being bullied at the local Safeway store. They both came up to us and hugged us all. The young girl started to cry then as well. Sarah and I started to cry as we just held each other so tight. This little lady was still in her Safeway uniform. She looked at me and once I looked at her I knew her from the day in the checkout line. She told her parents who I was and that I was the one who had helped her at work one day. I had helped her at work with a nasty man who was a bully. They hugged me harder and her mother whispered to me, "You have now saved both my daughters from harm." Sarah looked into my eyes and it warmed up my heart to feel such love and caring from people that mattered to me more than my soul's existence.

We ended up staying for around an hour and we told the family how we saved her and how she was such a fighter. The other crew had come into the room as well as the emergency resident that had pitched in and helped strip out and clean our unit. We slowly made our way out and had a look into our now stripped and clean unit. Some of the other staff came over and showed their support. They would take our unit, strip and wash it, make it ready for a call as soon as possible but it was not our responsibility today. We'd both had more than enough life saving for the one day. We both had seen too much blood. We wore more blood on us today then we should have in a lifetime of EMS. Looking back, we could not have had a better team to save a life.

It was clear that our success was due to the team that had worked so hard to save a life. My lifelong success was because of our winning team. Somehow, I needed to see that our real success knowing that the one part people will never forget about us was our efforts and how hard we worked as a team. Today we all gave 150% and it paid off. Nothing in general we did today was on our own. My friends from ER came out to the bay as they got time and gave me a hug. I then realized I was not going home. Someone had triaged me and I was seeing my friend once more today. I guess I had a longer visit with an emergency doctor than I had expected. He was more than a little worried about me. I on the other hand was not as worried as I knew in my heart I was in the safest place in the world. They on the other hand would not take a chance in letting me be alone tonight at home.

Apparently, I had a room reserved for me tonight. They were going to make sure I was not left alone tonight for any reason. I was taken to a private room and they grabbed me some hospital scrubs. Then my nurse smiled at me and said, "It's shower time." One of my closest friends in nursing made sure I was okay and they found me some real soap and some OR betadine scrub brushes. It was not until then that I realized I was covered in blood – it was soaked through my uniform and dried on in so many places. I showered forever trying to get the blood off. I had waited a little too long and it was caked on. But water and soap washed it all away. I just hoped I wasn't washing off the life she needed. She needed every drop of fluid we gave her. I was never scared of blood but to see it outside of someone so little that needed it was too much for me to handle.

When it was over I got dressed and went to lay down. I was exhausted. I had Tinsel and Pebbles waiting for me in the room on my bed. My other crew had gone to my place and snuck them into the hospital with the nurse's permission of course. We held each other for an hour. Tinsel tried to lay inside me. Pebbles just stretched out and went to sleep. They lay on both sides of me and Tinsel made sure everyone that came into the room was a good person. Pebbles just lay beside me and slept. Pebbles simply relied on Tinsel to keep watch. That evening I had every staff member I knew come in and make sure I was okay. They all gave me a hug from the heart and they took some of my pain away even if they didn't know they left with it, for now it was inside them too. Then one of the nurses brought in an extra stretcher. Sarah presented herself in scrubs and was my roommate. She too had seen our ER doctor and was staying with me. She needed a long hot shower too. She too needed to wash off the life-giving blood from her as well. Even angels can have some hard days I was now seeing.

Both puppies were asleep taking up some space on each bed. It was then I realized for the first time we were still supposed to be on shift for another two nights. I guess I had an unplanned holiday. I realized we were both off for the right reasons. We both needed to be off and we needed each other. Some of our friends could see that we needed each other more than ever tonight. I needed her more than she ever needed me it seemed. Sometime before midnight we just sat and looked at the ceiling and both could feel the love for each other. More than that, the level of respect was paid for in sweat and now with more blood than you could ever imagine.

For the next twenty-four hours, we were a family of one. Around midnight the staff physician came by and gave us some good news. When I saw him coming I thought the worst but prayed for the best. When he said, "She made it, that little girl made it," I was alive again. He said, "It will take time but they're hopeful of a full recovery." I was given something more positive that I needed, more than oxygen or breathing. I needed it more than light. Sarah and I held each other until I went to sleep. As soon as I had gone off to sleep I woke up trying to stop the bleeding again. Why would she still keep bleeding? I was pleading to myself to hurry up and stop it before it was too late. It was too much blood. There was just too much blood.

In seconds Sarah had me looking at her with a calm voice and suddenly I was okay. I was shaking. My heart was beating out of my chest. I was so scared and with a long hard hug and her reassuring words I came back to reality. Sarah was going to make me come back. Suddenly I was back to being in the hospital again. I was back to the right place and to the right time. One of the nurses also showed up at the right time and she passed me some pills and said, "Take these." I took them and closed my eyes again. I could still see the blood running off the stretcher. But I could hear the helicopter flying in hot and fast and it gave me hope. I could feel Sarah's heart beating against me as I held her tight. Thankfully I had someone to make sure I was safe and would get me through the longest, worst night after the worst call in a long time. With the sound of her heart beating and her easy breathing I went to a better place. I was safe. The world around me could not harm me. I was reassured she was okay and soon I could close my eyes again.

For hours, I dreamed and floated in a warm place in time. After that night, I was going to be okay. I didn't wake up for over twelve hours – it was in the late afternoon of the next day after our call. Sarah kept guard and no one else was allowed in to wake me. The nurse also ensured no visitors, so I was not to be disturbed for any reason. I'm not sure what they gave me but when I woke up with Sarah at my side smiling. She was reading her IPad. I was so thankful that some of my friends had taken the puppy's home sometime earlier but I didn't remember any of it. Somehow, I felt brand new. It was the first time in a very long time I felt good with myself. Somehow, I had needed a chemical-induced holiday. I also needed the mental break and it was what was needed to get me back up. That last call had taken its toll on me even if it still worked out in a positive way. Thank god for sending Sarah to keep me safe and for bringing me back from hell.

Our day crew showed up with my favourite Timmy's and some breakfast wraps when I was finally awake. It was later in the day but they knew they were my favourite. That hit the spot. My puppies always got the bacon. When I saw them both walk in, I knew I had the best EMS friends in the whole wide world. The biggest part about being on the right team was to know we mattered to each other 24/7 and even more. The fact that we always respected our partners and respected our other crews regardless of their level of training or their years of service; they still made up our team. We were so much more productive as a team. When we were a team we were unstoppable.

Thankfully I had my partner to keep me going. Our other crews were also amazing and we all helped each other out anytime possible just as they covered for us for the last two days. Over the last forty-eight hours our crews had gone over the top and made our lives bearable, despite the bad times we have faced over the years. The bad things all affect us at different times. Staff can have peaks and lows when they can cope better and days when they have had just enough before the burst. Some days it simply all adds up. Regardless of the bad some on our team helped and they changed a bad day to be a better day. They all mattered to me more than words could ever express. I could have simply gone home after my bad day but the interventions at the right time, by the right people, made the outcome so much more productive. The fact I was a patient and medicated at the right time saved me from another night of hell. With Sarah staying at my side throughout the darkness of the night the demons from hell never had a fighting chance. My avenging angel could not be cornered or assaulted this night. Tonight, I mattered to many people and that had to count for more than anyone would ever know.

Suddenly I realized just how important I was and just how everyone really matters to someone else. Once you realize it's the team effort that saves the lives, you will then value the input from the team members even more on every call. You then treat the team members more as equals, regardless of who they are or what their current level of education or training they've obtained. If only all EMS staff could also bond with their partners better we could enhance our level of care. I know if we treated students as part of our team over the years, our profession had a chance to survive.

As we lay in the hospital bed my body floated up and down from the air action to prevent pressure points. I thought about the last many days all rolled into just one. I just realized we needed to respect our newer co-workers more and give them the same chances we had to be successful in our own career. The last two days proved to me our team was perfect, despite the most stressful events. We had many good days and only rarely a bad day. But on our worst days they were the ones that mattered the most.

If it was not for each member helping each other we could not survive through the worst days of our lives. I knew Sarah had made my life so much better despite our very difficult calls and we completed the most challenging situations. We were going to be friends for life. We were also going to be EMS partners for life as well. We would get past this week and build our lives back up and sooner rather than later we would be responding to calls again. I was looking forward to it but also almost terrified or scared at the same time. Only Sarah would know my worst fears and my secret was always safe with her. More importantly, I could count on her to save my life. Just as I would do anything possible to keep harm away from her as well.

Brent - One of my true loyal friends.

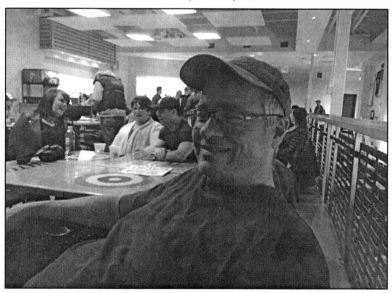

"We all support each other in more ways than we can ever see"

Chapter 21: Getting Back Up
"The Right Reasons"

The time to walk away is different for everyone in our profession. Every career has its peaks and lows. Every career has its starting points, it's advances and it also needs the right conclusion. The end of my EMS career for me would be on my terms. In many careers, you could plan to work until you were sixty-five but not in our profession. The unique thing about EMS is it's mentally, physically and emotionally taxing on anyone working the streets. Yes, we can all try to reduce our stress and continue to be physically active but our bodies can't take a beating forever. Past a certain point our body says it's had enough.

Working EMS doing emergency responses is not a nine to five job. Some will go that route but for some of us it's not even an option. I was never meant to work in an office. I was made to respond and help others on the scenes or wherever we were called. That life was the only life I knew. Some people are meant to be office people and some are politicians – I was neither. Sadly, what takes its toll is the long fourteen-hour shift; when for many reasons, you can't get enough sleep or rest between the shifts. Then you add a few sixteen-hours and then occasionally a thirty-six-hour marathon and it's just too much. The push to exceed your physical, mental and endurance limits comes to all of us some day.

We can take time away from the job, we can go on holidays and we can continue to seek support from our peers but there comes a time when our best is most often not good enough. I actually think my message to walk away after being knocked down one too many times came from an old TV show. I was watching a re-run of "Men in Black" (MIB), which came out around 1997. I got back up and was ready to battle the beast again but as Kay says in the movie MIB so well, "Once you have been inside a bug once you don't want to go back in." It was a good analogy to me to realize there comes a time when you don't want to see the worst of the worst anymore. There comes a time when you should be able to walk away knowing you have done your share of good deeds. Then you can pass the work onto the next generation and that is that.

After a lifetime of badness, I realized it was now Sarah, Robin and Ken's world to save. They are some of the best I had seen and now they were able to carry on my legacy. The last pediatric code was my signal. I took some time off after my short stay in the hospital. Call it a breakdown or crash and burn, I really don't care as my close friends and I know I had just gone too far one time too often. Thankfully I had my special friends and they brought me back from a hell that you can't explain unless you've been there. Not one person that found me in the bay crying soaked in a kid's blood will ever judge me harshly. They too will not forget that scene for a lifetime. Several of them went home and held their kids or spouse and cried one more time.

If you polled the rescuers and hospital staff on that call many would risk their life to save her as well. Some actually did during the initial time and transport, just as did the STARS crew, had done. Anyone working risked so much to help save a life of a precious child. Many staff went above and beyond to save her and that was all that needed to be said.

They had found me so broken and destroyed that I had nothing left to give. They pulled me back from hell and supported me as though I was the only one that mattered. That was what it took to bring me back. They shared my pain that day which was from a thousand bad calls. After that day, I was not the same. Sarah knew that and she watched me more closely. My friends from the RCMP and the fire services also supported me after that day. They stopped in and often checked in on me. They took me for coffee. They sat with me when I needed someone to support me the most. They showed me that our lives mattered to each other. That was what mattered to me.

After I had been back to work for several months I was still having some hard days. Today we were at the ninth-hour that had started normally and we had some fun but thankfully easy calls. Sarah and I took turns attending and she had just received confirmation to attend paramedic school and was registered to start in just over a month. She was sad and also glad about it as we had built such a bond we did not consider it work anymore. Thankfully she was granted an educational leave and she had been guaranteed a position as soon as she had finished "medic school" so it was a win-win for her. We had talked a lot recently about how our bond had grown and how we had both benefitted from each other in more ways than anyone could ever know or understand. I had saved Sarah and she had saved me on more than one occasion so we were family for life.

After the transfer, we had a little break in emergency calls and went to the city on a stat transfer. We decided to head to Timmy's at the end of our day on the way home from the city transfer. I suggested we get some food as we were off shift soon and then we could go home right after work and get some well-earned sleep. It was too late for us to do a call or we would be on overtime. They had a crew waiting and ready for the unit when we got home anyway. We had a busy but good shift. At one point, we had laughed so hard I almost I fell over. I told Sarah if I laughed hard enough to die, just let me go. I didn't think I could still laugh that hard. Sarah brought the best back out of me when I was a lost soul.

Thankfully, I had not forgotten how to laugh. It was still inside of me. Nothing could kill my ability to laugh with my real friends. We got a breakfast wrap and a large French Vanilla, as I needed the sugar rush and the internal caffeine support to keep my heart working at least for a few more hours. We sat down inside the store and I was bugging Lindsay who had just finished her Health Care Aide program to now become a registered nurse (RN) instead; then she could look after me when I was old and grumpy. She gave me a Gibbs slap to the back of the head in fun and said that I could never be old and grumpy. We were quietly eating, sipping away and I looked at Sarah and said, "I'm done, my friend." This is your last day of work, as it is my last day as well. Sarah never said much but sat and slowly finished her breakfast. Then she looked into my eyes and said, "Thank you." I was not sure what to say, so I never said anything. Then she made my career complete in her most sincere and honest words.

She spoke from her heart with more wisdom than I could ever imagine in any one person. Sarah stated, "You have given your life for others for more than most people would or could imagine. You have given your all from your heart even when you had nothing left to give. Many have not even given a third of your time in the industry or to the profession. The lifespan of most EMS professionals is around eight years so don't feel bad – you have given 400% more than most in just time alone. Looking at your lifetime of personal service tells more than most people could ever dream of knowing. You have probably seen more situations and complications that are not even in the EMS teaching books than they normally list in the library of medical complications or concerns. You don't owe this profession anything." I looked at her smiling and said, "You're probably right."

"You have seen the changes over three decades of healthcare with the good and the bad changes." I looked into her eyes and could see the sincere friendship and the loyalty that most partners never are able to achieve. In our short time, we had been to many calls together. We had seen a side of hell that only a select few would have to face. But most days we got to see the good side of people. We took our time and we treated people just a little more special than most for a good reason. They were all special to us for so many reasons. We had laughed and we had cried together with many. We had worked so well together we developed a bond that only a few partners could ever hope to achieve."

Together we broke the speed limits and we deviated from protocols so often my supervisors gave up trying to reprimand me at all anymore. They would just add them to my pile and that was all that needed to be said. The supervisors had seen us work and knew if we deviated from protocol it was for a valid reason. They also understood why and what we were speeding for or why we would take the calculated risk to speed.

The day we had the RCMP driving our unit we got about five speed alerts with a heavy police escort so I think it was justified. We actually cared too much instead of caring too little. There are many people alive or have lived longer and better because of us always working as a team. Sarah looked into my eyes and simply but sincerely said, "I would not be alive without your actions." I just sat and looked into her eyes and felt her heart but never said anything as I listened to her soothing voice and let my mind go back to many random events. I remembered the pure disasters we arrived at and we made it out alive with patients that now had a second chance. The patients I had talked to after they had been in cardiac arrest or intubated was something no one could take away from me for as long as time was on my side, they were still our wins. Only god knows the real difference we made in the big picture.

Our coffee break had gone on for a lot longer than I actually realized. It was the support needed to walk away with pride and dignity. I typed up my resignation letter as Sarah drove us back to our base. As we backed into the hall I wasn't sure I could send it. I asked Sarah to read it and she did so right away. Then in a split second she pushed the send button and shut my phone off. It was done. I could now walk away. I had to walk away on my terms, but I needed the extra help to make it happen. I could not have been able to send it and Sarah knew that. Now we had four more tours together and we would be free. We planned our coffee date for later that day after we'd had some sleep. Somehow fate was with me and I was not at war with anyone or anything but my inner pain which was bearable.

We went in and signed off our drugs and ensured our unit was cleaner and better than when we started. We moved a few things around in the kits to make sure the next crew knew just how much we loved them. We added some toys to see if the next crew was awake when they did the unit check. They would smile when they found our little pranks and they too would put the toys somewhere else for us on our first day back. It's something we did just to make sure they knew we loved and cared for them and that too mattered.

The drive home was so fulfilling. I took my time. I looked at the scenery and I made sure I didn't go my normal route that day. I wanted to drive the roads I had never travelled going to or from work. I stopped at a small hardware store on the way home and went in and purchased a few random items. The one thing I really wanted was a nice outdoor patio rocker made out of real wood. Thankfully, they had a few books that had some good ideas. I would purchase what I needed over the next few days and I'd make my own rocker. In my world "If you needed something built right you would just do it yourself," I was so commonly fond of saying. I needed a hobby and I needed to make sure I was not alone in the days to come. For the last part of my EMS career I had the most loyal companions in the world waiting for me every day. I could leave and forget something and when I walked in the door they were in heaven all over again. They never let me down.

This day I got off work I was feeling okay. I took Pebbles and Tinsel for a good long run and then we slept for as long as they would let me. After, we got up and sat on the back deck and decided what was next in my life. I was trying to think of how to change the world for the good or make it better. I had seen so much tragedy and stupidity to last me for a lifetime and I wanted to help change the future for our kids. I texted Sarah and said: "meet me in an hour at Timmy's". I was hoping Lindsay was working to see her big smile and to bug us. We would bug her back. In fifteen seconds, the response was simply "10-4." I took the killers for a walk and thought about it some more. How could we change the world to be better than it was? The answer was that it had to come from the children or from our younger generation of leaders and that was the only way. Most politicians and leaders were not normally into redesigning a world to improve it but rather for personal or other self-serving commitments. Many had no desire to change the world but ensure they were popular or being rewarded in status or financially.

Most people don't see the world as a disaster, as they didn't see our perspective from day to day. They don't work night shift with us and they don't have a clue how bad the streets are for so many unfortunate people. We see the worst of the worst 24/7. The police see it much worse and they are in a terrible situation where the legal system has fallen apart in all different directions. The money and the power struggles corrupt so many systems. So, we had to find a way to circumvent the future for our children and somehow or someway they could change the future, was my inner thoughts. Somehow, I wanted our future to change for we had the technology and the wisdom but for some reason we never had the long-term vision that was needed to change the world to be a better place for all of us.

After meeting with Sarah, I told her my idea. She thought about it while we sat and watched the world go past. Then she said, "We can always just get the system to add First Responder and the Emergency Medical Responder to the current school curriculum." I said, "Do you think anyone would listen?" Sarah said, "Let's try. We have nothing to lose and millions of lives to help or to try to save. We can at least try." "Why not?" I replied. "Okay let's try and meet with the School Board and get a meeting with the right people and bring up our ideas." All we have to lose is an idea and that cost us nothing.

Sarah said she would call and arrange it and she would make a presentation to go along with it. After it was done she would send it to me for review. "Sounds like a good plan," I told her. We finished our friendly planning session and said good-bye for the day. We both had some things to do and sleep was one more thing on our to do list waiting for both of us. Overall, I thought it was a solid idea. It would help students be more responsible, it would teach them all real-life skills and it would let them see a side of caring and compassion that many had not seen in the past. Just maybe it would curb down some of the alcohol use and abuse, as well help lessen the street drug abuse incidents, and eventually lessen the driving while distracted incidence in our younger drivers. We had some good ideas if only we had a chance we could at least try to help the world.

Maybe we could make a difference if we taught people at the right age the reasons why certain behaviours were wrong. We needed to start somewhere and our kids were the only solution I could see if it was ever possible. After I read a USA Drug Enforcement Agency article about the fentanyl crisis where they claimed the US had about 700 deaths in 2014 and by the end of 2015 they had over 13,000 deaths. Then in 2016 it had soared up to 50,000 people. That made me think teaching the kids was the right thing to do as well as make First Responders or EMR a high school elective. Thinking about our busy days it was no wonder the EMS services were getting overrun with drug-abuse-related emergencies.

Hopefully our actions would help decrease the impaired driving rates that the First Responder and the EMR courses actually can touch or in some way provide a form of deterrent. Hopefully people could see it was killing too many people. Our legal system would not like it as many lawyers are making money from trying to defend the guilty drunk drivers to allow them to continue driving drunk over and over.

Just lately the manufacturing of the Alcohol Ignition Interlocking System could not be produced in a large enough quantity in the province of New Brunswick which tells me it's a serious problem, if nothing else in that province for sure. While reading the MADD Canada web site they claimed in 2012 that about fifty-eight percent (58%) of the crashes were from alcohol use or abuse. Sadly, that is about 1500 deaths a year. Plus, there are many more hurt as well as many more innocent people killed and hurt from its effects. We had to push our hidden agenda for what it was worth. Somehow, we had to challenge the world to be a better place to live. We had to find a way to lesson the plea bargaining and let the system be a real deterrent to the real crimes.

Our next tour started with a great surprise. Ken was back and had just done his EMR course. Ken wanted to do a ride-along with us this tour and get some extra experience and we both said, "Sure why not?" We talked to our supervisor "Greg" and it was approved in seconds. Ken would ride out with us for our last four tours. Then he would be off to EMT Primary Care Paramedic school. I think it was amazing, as it was a way out for both us to enjoy our job but to also teach someone we both knew and we believed in. Ken would distract us and we could give 110% until our very last call. I could not think of a better way to finish off my career. I would not admit it, but my back was killing me. My knees and my right ankle were also not happy carrying people up or down the stairs anymore. I'd give anything for a two-hour stint in a hot-tub most days after work. I just had to keep walking for another month and then crawling would be also an option. Wheelchairs were for seniors and I was no senior, minus the grey hair and the lifetime of physical, mental and personal abuse. Somehow, I would keep going. Quitting was not an option. Crawling kept you from falling hard enough to have an intracranial bleed if you needed a reason to be low to the ground.

Our first call this tour was for a choking person with chest pain. It sounded like a strange call but we had not much to go on from our dispatch information. It was either a breathing problem or a cardiac-related call. My strange habit of building a solid list of differential diagnosis as well as thinking about the common "H&Ts" which were Hypoxia, Hypovolemia, Hypoglycemia, or Trauma, Tablets and Thrombosis which was commonly seen in the heart making it a cardiac event, or related to the brain or pulmonary systems. There were others but these were the common complications we always considered. My brain was already working double time. I would just think about the worst thing we needed to rule out and the rest was optional.

I was thinking this is close to a small community and we were the closest unit but we had no backup easily available today. So, our second-best option was to send the local volunteer firefighters and made sure we had more immediate medical backup en route. They could apply the oxygen, give ASA, and could start CPR if needed. If possible, they would get us a medical history and much more. They would ensure we had easy access to the patient and would assist us in loading our patient as well. In the worst-case scenario, they could even drive for us, even if it was bending our operational rules as it often happened. We had them dispatched right after we were on the road just to be on the safe side. Plus, they would help us with extrication if it was a difficult extrication due to stairs or because of the patient's size and weight. Often getting patients out of a residence was a small nightmare.

We were about eight minutes from the scene when our dispatch updated us and I started to laugh and we were also a little embarrassed. The patient was apparently in chronic pain, had taken a big drag on his illegal marijuana and then fainted. The dispatcher would also be laughing as the firefighters were now on scene and our scene was considered secured. Smoke is not an issue now – just a residual sedating smell I would say. I guess the firefighters can at least make sure the house is ventilated a little before our arrival. It would be a good time for the police to stop for a visit but we would not call them.

As we started slowing down to enter the community I said to Ken, "This is your call – we are your backup. Just have fun and if you have any questions, ask. It will just be like school only not a simulated patient." I said, "Just remember if he passes out, just start CPR, but only do "chest compressions" until he looks into your eyes and then it will all be good. If he's faking it you will know right away and if not, we will be applying the monitor and getting ready to defibrillate him." The airway is optional at least for the first minute in most cases of adult cardiac arrest.

As we pull up we parked by the side door of the house, we grabbed our kits and follow Ken in with Sarah going to look after Ken. I will just there to bug the firefighters and get the scene history. Ken is greeted by four smiling volunteer firefighters and is escorted to the patient. He is on the floor with a pillow propped up behind his head. He looks to be in a confused state and he is not focusing on us very well. Ken reached for a pulse and quietly said, "20-30 bpm at the wrist." I think Sarah was also shocked and she too reached for a pulse. Then she rapidly applied the monitor and said, "Well, Houston, we have a problem." That got my attention. Sarah said, "It looks to be a second-degree type 2 AV block and also a third-degree heart block at times as well. I will grab a 12-lead right now. Can you start an IV, grab a blood sugar and also a quick temperature to rule out sepsis?" I said, "Sure." Ken and I got that done right away. I also did a quick head to toe examination and could see a malnourished middle-aged gentleman about sixty years old who looked to have had a hard life. Some people have never been dealt a fair hand in life. We would never know how he ended up in this moment in his life but we would not judge or refuse him care for any reason. Today he was our only concern and he mattered more than most as he was ill and needed us despite the recreational drug use or abuse.

As my partners did the basic care I was looking at his medication containers and getting the volunteers firefighters' verbal report. They found him in his chair, unresponsive. They quickly picked him up and slid him to the floor and were going to start CPR right away. One of them was also applying the AED and as they were pushing the analyze button his eyes slowly opened up. They had almost started CPR but one of their staff is LPN at the local senior's lodge and she told them to wait a minute. Sure enough, he started coming to a little more and life was coming back after they laid him down. Regardless of the AED interpretation or electrical generated thought to shock or not shock they simply just shut it off. If he was dead or looked dead a shock would not hurt. Today a shock to his heart was not a priority.

After they knew he was alive they put his feet up and applied the oxygen with a NRB face mask, as his oxygen saturation was lower than 80% on room air; the oxygen level came up rapidly as his breathing rates were adequate. Then they just needed our help. For that they knew we were coming in hot and fast. They would be smiling more as we pulled outside. Thankfully he was breathing, but not well. In no time, his oxygen saturation had picked up but the heart rate stayed very slow, with a BP that was really low around 60-70 systolic by palpation. They had tried a few times but it was not easy to get a good BP as it was so low.

Essentially, he was in cardiogenic shock but we were not sure why. I said to Sarah and Ken, "Let's just grab him and go to the unit and start to work." Sarah was applying the pacing pads right away after the 12-lead was obtained. This residence was a big mess and it's safer and better to go to the unit as soon as possible in all cases so I said, "Let's just go to our office and then we can get to work," and Sarah nodded in agreement. I hope you don't mind, Ken, but Sarah is taking over and I'm her servant today. She just laughed at me and said, "Call our friends from the sky and see if they want to fly." I said, "As you wish, my princess," and walked outside for better phone reception and to clear my head from the sedating odour. Funny for right now I was completely numb.

I think I was already legally impaired. In less than a minute we had a STARS chopper moving to the local landing pad and was initiating a "priority one" launch sequence. The staff were preparing to come to our rescue as soon as they could get airborne. We would not be waiting in the city hallways today for an Interventional Cardiac Catheter lab or an ICU bed. So, all in all it was a win-win for both our services. They were also bringing a physician who could feed a special pacing wire in if our external pacer was ineffective. We had our bases covered.

We had firefighters already moving to set up a landing pad at a local good wide and open intersection. The local RCMP also arrived and would ensure the scene was dealt with. They helped the firefighters set up a secure landing zone. Today they were another part of the team; charges or concerns of the drugs are not a concern when you're worried about saving a life. They would kindly notify the next of kin for us as well. I was sure the evidence would just have got destroyed and that would be that. This man had enough problems in his life right now than to worry about his chronic pain habits. Today our patient just needed to stay alive and we would look after the rest.

In no time, we had him to the unit and we attacked him. We set up the monitor to do the BP every five minutes. A CO_2 detector was added to the nasal prongs and we switched the mask to our NP/CO_2 detector to 4 LPM and the oxygen saturations that maintained his oxygen saturation over 94% so we were all happy. Sarah noticed the blood sugar was low and after she got an IV started she would start an IV bolus and give half an ampule of dextrose slowly as well. The temperature was 36.8 degrees celsius so it was normal but maybe warmer than I would expect so it would bear some watching as well.

We all agreed we needed an advanced airway for transport. The Online Medical Director (OLMC) as well as the STARS physician agreed. I drew up some Ketamine and I then injected 1 mg/kg and started to get ready to initiate the artificial pacemaker. The BP was too low for any other medications. We started at a pacing rate of 60 bpm and slowly raised the pacing power until it captured. At about 60 milliamperes (mA) we had electrical and mechanical capture. The IV bolus was running and the lungs were dry so we kept adding the fluid as the patient looked very dry. Being he was altered, the pacing never really bothered him much and the Ketamine took his mind to a better place so it was a win-win. As they paced him I intubated him with Heather my firefighter helper at my side. God her smile ensured my day would always be golden no matter our patient's outcome.

As soon as we had the pacing started and the heart rate showing mechanical and electrical capture, I was much happier. I was hanging the Dopamine while Sarah and Ken were trying for a second IV line. It would be our backup in case we lost our primary IV site, which happens from time to time. Most likely they would insert a central line in CCU or ER but for now we could give our emergency fluid access site. It would also work with a triple lumen adaptor for IV medication and physiological or chemical pressors peripherally for now. After a one litre bolus of normal saline, the BP was up to 82/38 so it was a little better but the MAP was not good enough so we added the Dopamine at 5 mcg/kg/min and would titrate as needed. STARS updated us they would be down beside us in about ten minutes and we were ready for them. Today they were our rapid transport and hopefully they would have an uneventful flight if you called pacing, IV infusions, cardiac interventions and ALS uneventful. Sadly, if this was some of the services we knew, not much at all would be done – that was just the norm and no one even cared.

I then was ready to have some fun and tried to get Ken feeling more at home in our unit. I said to Ken, "Now you're in charge again. What should we do now, my friend?" He thought about it and then he just winked at me. "Ask Sarah, Sarah will know." I laughed out loud. He was a very fast learner. Although she was only registered as an EMT-A (Primary Care Paramedic - PCP) she was solid in her BLS and also her ALS care. She would be bored with some of the classes as she had already studied way more than most I had ever seen but that was to keep me out of trouble I would expect.

Sarah was more than ready for paramedic school. That was the best place for her next education adventure although she should seek a higher or greater goal if time and her education were fair to her. She would make a great emergency physician if she got the chance to make it to that level. Her dreams would let her fly to her goals. I would help her anyway possible for as long as I was alive, she could count on me.

I sat back and thought about our call. Then I thought about a good point to bring up with Ken. Call it a teaching point or just the right time to pass on a little wisdom from a lifetime of helping people. I said to Ken, "Don't be afraid to change the world with the things that we can help change. Ken, you can become anything you want to be and with the right attitude you will and can change the world around you. Make everyday a challenge to help people and somehow over time you will change the world." I said, "Ken, become a paramedic, or better yet become an emergency physician and you will make the difference in many more lives." This call had made me realize just how well calls could go. Even when we had serious issues they were easily fixed.

Today, we showed Ken that despite the team around us, we all could be part of the team. When you push people to be the best they can be, they will excel in everything they try to achieve. When we display integrity and honesty to our co-workers, we show that our efforts are valiant despite the outcomes. When we try our hardest despite the challenges or the difficulties we face, we are rewarded by the effort in many ways. Our co-workers, our patients and the patients' families will see the efforts we are putting into helping others and it is rewarded with gratitude more often than we expect most days.

Today we got back our ability to work hard, have fun, save a life and take time to help our newest EMS member be part of a team. To us both that was the greatest day possible. We had been knocked down and had many bad events but this call had given us strength to get back up. We did our job and we made someone else's life count even if he was having a bad time. Today he got a second chance and hopefully cardiology, the pain clinic, the internal medicine specialist and the modern aspects of our medicine system will give him a better outlook on life. Today he would get a second chance and he was worth it to us all.

We watched STARS coming in from the west of our location coming to us high and fast. In no time, they were circling and setting up for an inline approach to our prepared landing zone. Today our firefighters, the RCMP and our crew had made a potential bad outcome a good outcome. Tonight, we could all sleep better despite the crazy feeling or buzz from the recreational smoke that lingered on all of us for the rest of the shift. That was the least of our worries today. Today we had a good day.

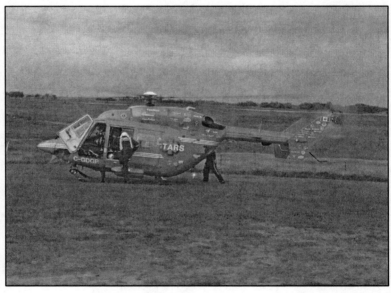

"Helping or saving one person at a time"

"True Friends Matter"

I never dreamed this day would come but one day I woke up and just like that, I knew I was done. I knew the day I was not able to give 110% I had to walk away. I had seen many others that stayed too long and they became bitter and unproductive members in our EMS or healthcare world. I thought more about how to leave over the next few weeks and I had to resort to sitting down with a few close friends to make a plan that was unique to me for walking away. I looked back at my career and needed to know I had completed my task. I wanted to ensure I had made a difference in others' lives and my lifelong work was completed for some strange reason. I had so many thoughts but no real answers for some time in this part of my life. I looked back and wondered about my success stories but my regrets also came to the surface. I had many personal and professional regrets about my decisions over the years but I had assumed the consequences of my decisions whether there was a good or bad outcome.

I wanted to know I could walk away with no regrets in the timing of my walking away. I needed to know if I could sleep knowing I did my best, despite the outcomes. The only way to walk away is to leave a legacy to help my friends keep going even when I was not able to be at their side. I decided it was time to take my partner for coffee a month ago, and together with some advice from someone I trusted with my life. I would make a plan to walk away. Knowing that was the first step but how to walk away and not leave a hole in my soul or cause others grief or suffering was my primary goal. Sarah had actually helped plan my walking away.

She understood my pain and she knew with her leaving for school I would get a new partner. I told her "she was and would also be my last EMS partner." I had seen several newer staff members that had come to our service and were not respectful of some senior staff. Some were lazy and some were in EMS for the wrong reasons. I knew that was my sign to leave. It was time to pack up my wonderful golden retrievers and head east until I found an ocean and a parking stall with my name on it. It was just my time. I was stopping to see Don and Sally as well as the kids on the way past. Their golden retriever puppies were now big enough to be the protectors of the three little ladies and that made me so proud to know they were safe and protected. Sarah would miss me but she would always have a key and a ticket to come visit at anytime.

I looked back at the stressful calls over the last months, the years and the decades and I knew it was the right time. I had slowly lost the ability to keep the calls organized, to intervene and think at the speed I demanded from myself. The skills were easy but the motions or my dexterity were not as good. Some things were getting harder. One of the biggest examples I noticed was I was having a little more trouble with my ability to starting an IV now-a-days. It was not as easy as it had been for thirty or more years anymore. I also noticed a slight tremor starting in my right arm; even though it was slight it was still not a good sign. I didn't want to be told to retire as my whole life was on my terms. My whole life I had fought my battles and taken my losses with grace. I wonder if it was God's way of saying to me it was time to walk away gracefully, all while I still had a reason to live. I still could appreciate the outdoors and I had many more trips planned to see the quiet and peaceful parts of the world that needed my supervision. I would retire with my famous golden retrievers and ensure they were spoiled for as long as I was blessed to have them in my life. After all, how many golden retrievers have ridden in fire trucks, they also had ridden in ambulances, or had been on multiple road trips around the province checking on EMS students? They were the true heroes for saving my life more than once.

My biggest reason was easy to see as it was the best pair of golden retrievers in the whole world who adored my every second with them. They were slowly getting older but so was I, we were a good aging team. My only regret was not having someone to bug or to spoil but that was most likely for the best just as well. I would never want to share my pain and my sleepless nights with anyone else. Maybe it was the best overall outcome that no one had to share my pain. My two golden retrievers understood and knew when I was having my bad days and on a bad day they were closer. They never left me alone.

On a good day, they did their own thing but still kept me in sight. Even when I had to go to the bathroom one of them always followed. It was a good thing I was not embarrassed having them watching me have a shower or soak in the tub, as they just made sure I was safe. They thought I needed them more than they needed me, I think. They were the best and most loyal companions I could ever hope for in my life.

Thinking back to my worst days, they knew even before I got home. They were more special or intuitive than most people I have ever known. They never asked if I was having a good or a bad day. They already knew the answer. After a really bad call I came home and the tears were in my eyes as I parked my truck. I got into the house and normally they would bark and make so much noise to tell me they were excited but this one-day they just let me in. They both jumped up on me and tried their best to hug me. I knew that day they were a blessing and they didn't get the lie I was okay, when they already knew it was a terrible day.

We sat there for a bit as I got my bearings and thoughts back together, got back into the truck and we went for a drive. We found a place to park just in the field of my Hutterite friends field. We all just sat and watched the world go past together. They were my debriefing tool for the hell from a bad shift when my partner was not around or when we could not unwind or debrief while at work or after the calls. Sometimes it was just not practical. They would not judge me for the good or the bad outcomes. Only once I could not get home and debrief with them but then they were brought to me for my therapy just the same. They had also done their time in a hospital healing me when needed.

It's truly amazing but animals know when you have internal pain or if you are suffering an illness. They know suffering and have the best addicting treatment for some of the most terrible events that life creates or passes out. They had one therapy that seemed to work very well – love. The love took the pure evil right out of my system and it just disappeared. I slowly understood the role of animals as therapy for PTSD over the years; to our pain and the inner turmoil it had created within many of us. The suffering was misunderstood on many levels and it was only recently people realized it was killing us all in record numbers. We needed to learn or assume the lessons our animals have taught us. Service dogs with all EMS, police, fire and especially military members with PTSD have been lifesaving on many occasions. The role of service dogs or other animals as pet therapy is still most likely not understood to its full extent.

In this modern age of technology, we need to learn how to forgive others even more. We need to learn to share our world in an unself-ish manner. We need to just take the time to help others in need when they need us the most. We need to support our friends more and not wait until it's convenient for us to help. We have all got so busy that many people miss the fact we have people in need all around us who were in trouble. I feel for the people in other countries having pure hell but let's care for our people first and ensure they are taken care of before they are lost. Somehow, we never even notice until we stop and look around and take the time to see the real world for what it is all around us. The people close to us should matter the most. We all need to remember to make today count for something everyday for the rest of our life. All I can ask is for you all to forgive me for needing to walk away.

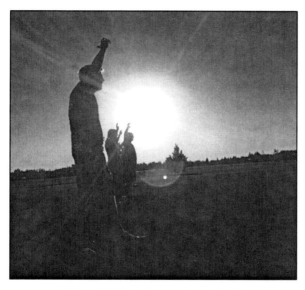

"Our EMS Family stands as One"

Conclusions Between Life & Death

Surviving the Darkness

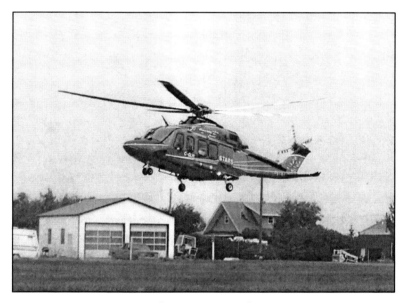

"All Lives Matter"

This book will take you all from the introduction of the current EMS service to some of the beginning early parts of my trials and tribulations throughout an active EMS career. On any ambulance call or with any patient transport you could never always predict an outcome, as things are constantly changing from all directions at the same time. Your patient could deteriorate or improve at anytime, you would have to find the best road to and from a call and you would also need to find a receiving hospital or a home for your sick and injured patients that is the most appropriate in the current condition or situation.

You would need to adapt to and overcome any situation as well as handle any possible complication all while doing patient care at a scene, during transport and finally on our arrival. You will be able to walk into our minds and see our thoughts as well as learn our innermost secrets. You will see the crews' intimate collaborative thoughts, see our personal struggles, and see the unique ways of helping thousands of people in need or in distress. It simply shows that we all have many good and some very bad days. The good and the bad days we have are all part of our line of work. No matter the calls we face, we face them as a team.

This book will show you through my eyes my daily wins as well as some of my personal struggles. On some of the worst days you will see just how hard life can be for a certain few unfortunate people. I will demonstrate what pure strength, endurance, as well as hope contributes to the patient's' ability to live. There will be people who will defy the laws of physics – they face death and refuse to die and they will beat the ultimate odds. Along with their battle we will be at their side and not let them go. We will stand up for them when others look away. You will see, hear, smell and feel our every part to providing the best patient care possible.

Over time, this book will show you the courage required to face a new day, the ultimate dedication that comes from the heart, as well as the teamwork that is required for it all to happen. You will see the pure love received from helping others that sets the bar higher than most. Rarely, you will come across a few practitioners who give everything they have to help others in any situation and go above and beyond society's expectations. With the right crew at a sick or injured person's side, miracles can be made to happen. Life is too precious not to try harder than our personal limits.

In this book, you will have seen the love and the bond made between co-workers who share many personal challenges while working the ninety-six hours, always a team for the two days and two night shifts we worked together. We face the worst of the worst calls and then we will also do many easy or standard calls together where the interventions are minimal. Sometimes we are pushed until we are almost at our breaking point on certain calls. We often experience our bad calls back-to-back or in a short time frame. The best we can do is to monitor each other and help each other make it through the rougher days. I have your back and you have mine is the only way it can work.

On many calls or events, we have limited equipment as well as limited resources available. We often count on each other to carry us or help support our morale and also give each other spiritual help. Many days I just needed to just go on when I had nothing left but somehow my partner picked me up and made our day work. I slowly got to know how to defeat the odds and bend the rules enough to make my tour of duty count even more than anyone could ever imagine.

There is nothing in the world that is as challenging, emotional, stressful, and complicated as working EMS trying to save lives or by helping people in need. It is also a very rewarding sensation when you look back at a lifetime career in the Emergency Medical Services. Over the years, you will see many life and death challenges that will have good and tragic outcomes. There are no two days that will be the same.

The biggest challenges are the constant changes in medicine and EMS that never stop. The number of personal struggles, injuries, as well as the verbal and physical insults, along with the sleepless nights over the years is immeasurable. After some time, they were just expected. In the end, the rewards are not as frequent as you might expect but they always seem to just come at the right moment. When I compare the highlights of the good times to the bad times it's still worth the stress and the heartache. Looking back, so many of the events were mind-boggling or simply too complex to recall most people but we got through them all. The disasters, or the bad days somehow seem to all melt into one terrible day on our worst ones. This is when you just keep going ahead and don't look back.

You will see sudden cardiac deaths, respiratory emergencies, and simply the sick people that need a ride to a hospital. We will try to revive many and we will try to help or try to save many lives in danger. The biggest jobs you will do as a paramedic is lessen or decrease the personal suffering of many. The biggest reward we will most likely see is a few miracles from time to time. Being in EMS for most of my life I've seen many trends and changes in patient care. The biggest changes would be the modern era of electronics and the implementation of our designer drugs. When many of us started in the industry as an EMT or EMR it was without the use of the complex medications. Then over time to the end of my career as a paramedic I have seen many medications introduced to the emergency medical field. We have even seen the arrival of specialized medications designed for clot-specific cardiac or stroke disease. We have gone from guessing how medications worked to knowing exactly how the medications work at a cellular level. Even twenty years ago, we gave certain medications with no real idea of what they did but we admired the side effects just the same.

We have gone from getting generic directions over the phone such as "it's just north of the water tower" to learning how to read the county maps, then to being told where to go with the computer-aided dispatch (CAD's) in our units. We went from being on our own with no one really knowing where we were unless we radioed someone. We went from our nursing staff from our local hospital being our dispatcher to a satellite or telephone tower aided dispatch centre knowing where we are within a few hundred meters.

Now we are being dispatched and monitored 24/7 to our exact location and speed with a backup unit only one computer button away. They even know when we arrive on scene or when we are starting to transport, to our ultimate arrival at the receiving hospital. We actually went from landlines to VHF radios, then to cellular phones and finally to computer-aided dispatch systems where it is rare to talk to a dispatcher or a receiving hospital.

The human touch or the personal feeling of patient care has lessened somewhat over the last several years. Society has slowly decreased the level of caring about others, in my perspective. Our crews are seeing an increase in drug abuse, elder abuse and a lack of accountability overall in people. We've gone from having the sensation of caring or physical contact with patients to more like a robotic function of just going to work. Society forgot people mattered and our beliefs about helping others seemed not to matter as much anymore. Not every change is bad, as we can easily see from the many components of our job or career that life is better with the many positive changes.

One of the biggest changes in our career is the enhanced ability to be able to help people more in depth over time with modern medical expertise and equipment advances. With the increased wisdom obtained from past encounters, we have learned how to demonstrate and improve outcomes in certain treatments and with specific medications. It was almost like a teaching book that never stopped being edited. Just as I figured out the basic rules, someone changed the book again and before I knew it, changed it again.

The benefit was as we got the next level figured out we progressed to a higher level of care so it was always a positive climb up the wealth of wisdom. It was like a really old video arcade game that started easy and at every level became more and more challenging. In the end, we had the ability to perform every skill and know every shortcut but when I reached that level my body was ready for a retirement holiday. The changes are constant and the ever-changing world never stopped adapting to our care. Somehow, we made it work. Despite the challenges, we made it work for the best outcome possible.

We mastered the ability to multi-task in any situation. For years, we make the impossible happen but one day I realized I was running out of the right stuff. I tried to do my best for years but suddenly one day I noticed that something was not right anymore. I'd lost my personal edge. Without my edge, I can't give 110% anymore. I wasn't sure what the problem was but I knew I was seeing the world in slow motion and that wouldn't work. One day I was driving at my maximum speed and started getting suddenly very nervous. That made me realize that we all can only do this job for so long. Responding to people's emergencies and seeing many disasters I had reached my saturation point. One day I was the best of the best and the next day I was done. Just like that I lost my unique edge. If I was to live life on my terms I had to walk away before I made a mistake or cause personal harm.

Looking back that is how it slowly progressed, from a straightforward challenging career of saving lives and helping others, to an endless day. All of a sudden, I realized I had done my best for so long but today my best was not as good as it was yesterday. Once doubt starts to enter your brain, then you know it's time to walk away before you do harm. I could never live with those consequences. My whole career was trying to learn more and more. Be the best of the best. Everything we did over the years was to help people in need when they needed us the most.

I realized it's time for my partners to take over and it's time for me to make my exit on my terms. Slowly I found a way to make my exit, my final battle against the pain and suffering. I had fought it my whole life but the day came when I had to walk away and let others carry on the battle. I planned my last tour. I went in with as much energy as I could muster and walked away with my head held high. I walked away strong and proud knowing my legacy was my biggest achievement and also my personal reward.

As I drove away the sun was coming up and the birds were singing. The world was still within my grasp. Today is the day for me to go and make peace with the world from my backyard. Today I've earned the day off. My EMS friends will master my commitment and my many good friends and patients are in good hands. Many EMS families have each other to watch out for them in the EMS world and my personal guidance is now in their hearts, performed by their hands and seen in their daily practice to help others. A good quote comes to mind today as I walk away for the last time.

> *"Knowing when to walk away is wisdom."*
> *"Being able to is pure courage."*
> *Walk away, with your head held up high and be proud!"*

Author: Unknown

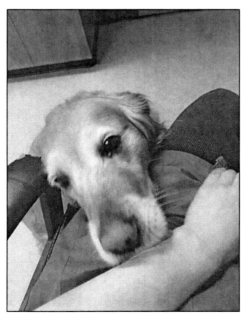

Dr. Natasha Borowski with Tinsel - "Your Spirit Will Never Die"

"Tinsel's love for life, love for freedom was right to the very end – for that was simply just my Tinsel!"

Closing Dedications to My Past Co-workers and the Best Role Models in the World

My dedication to the completion of "Between Life & Death: Surviving the Darkness" is to the most amazing people I've had the privilege to work with throughout my long EMS career. Every one of the people listed below is very precious to me and consistently helps to make my life better every day.

This book is a testament to my excellent partners throughout my long career in EMS through more stressful, demanding situations then you could imagine. There are too many to name. Along the way we made the world just a little bit better together as a team. The ones I've listed are all deserving of the real-life recognition that they so deserve.

- *Cathy Falconer RN* / U of A – Stollery Emergency Pediatric Trauma Coordinator / ATLS Course Coordinator / Friend for Life

- *Cheryl Cameron EMT-P* / Co-Instructor / ACLS / PALS Co-instructor / Former Beaver EMS Supervisor / Co-worker / Lifelong Friend

- *Dave Oleksyn EMT-A* / Tofield Fire Chief / Lifelong EMS Friend and EMS Partner

- *Debbie Smeaton* / Former Co-Director of Community Education & Manager of EMS Programs for Lakeland College / Lifelong Friend

- *Dr. Adrian Rothaney* / U of A – Stollery Emergency Physician

- *Dr. Alison Kabaroff-Berry* / Emergency Physician / AHS Medical Director

- *Dr. Bill Sevcik* / U of A – Stollery Emergency Physician / Educator / ACLS / PALS Medical Director / Friend for Life

- *Dr. Brian Rowe* / U of A – Stollery / Emergency Physician / Researcher / Educator

- *Dr. Chris Venter* / Wetaskiwin Health Centre / Emergency Physician / Family Physician

- *Dr. Christoff de Wet* / Wetaskiwin Health Centre / Emergency Physician / Family Physician

- **Dr. David Hoshizaki** / *U of A – ER / STARS / Emergency Physician*

  - **Dr. Eddie Chang** / *U of A – Stollery STARS / Emergency Physician / Educator / ACLS / PALS Medical Director* / Friend for Life

- **Dr. Erik Johnson** / *Wetaskiwin Health Centre / Emergency Physician / Family Physician*

- **Dr. Kevin Neilson** / *U of A – ER / STARS / Emergency Physician* / Friend for Life

- **Dr. Layton Burkhart** / *U of A – ER / STARS / Emergency Physician*

- **Dr. Leanda Stassen** / *Wetaskiwin Health Centre / Emergency Physician / Family Physician* / Friend

- **Dr. Mary Stephens** / *FRCSC / FACS / Clinical Professor / General Surgeon / Trauma Team Leader / Trauma Surgeon / ATLS Course Director / Critical Care Specialist*

- **Dr. Praveen Jain** / *Emergency Physician / Educator / ACLS / PALS / ITLS Medical Director* / Friend

- **Dr. Robert Broad** / *Neurosurgeon / ATLS Course Director / Trauma Team Leader / Critical Care Specialist*

- **Dr. Robin Arent** / *U of A – Stollery Emergency Physician / Pediatrician*

- **Dr. Samina Ali** / *U of A – Stollery / Emergency Physician / Pediatrician / Researcher* / Friend

- **Dr. Simon Ward** / *Wetaskiwin Health Centre / Emergency Physician / Family Physician*

- **Dr. Stiaan van der Walt** / *Wetaskiwin Health Centre / Emergency Physician / Family Physician*

- **Dr. Tuhin Bakshi** / *Wetaskiwin Health Centre / ACLS / PALS Co-instructor / Emergency Physician / Family Physician* / Friend

- **Dr. Yunus Moolla** / *Wetaskiwin Health Centre / Emergency Physician / Family Physician*

- **Elna Eidsvik, RN** / *Northern Nurse* / Friend for Life

- **George Stassen EMT-A** / *EMS Partner* / Lifelong Friend

- **Greg Vaal Pastor – EMT-P** / My Lifesaver

- **Heather Verbaas EMT-P** / *Past Student / Co-Instructor ACLS / PALS Co-instructor / ACP Staff* / Lifelong Friend

- **Kevin Fornel EMT-P** / *Fire Chief Viking Fire / Co-Instructor / ACLS / PALS Co-instructor* / Lifelong EMS Friend

- **Len Stelmaschuk EMT-P** / *Past Student / Co-Instructor / ACLS / PALS Co-instructor / Former Camrose EMS Manager / Beaver EMS Co-worker* / Lifelong Friend

- **Norm Martineau EMT-P** / *LPN / Past Student / ACLS / PALS Co-instructor* / Friend for Life

  - **Patricia Penton EMT-P** / *Keyano EMS Program Director*/ Lifelong EMS Friend & Coworker

  - **Rob Hastie EMT-P** / *Past Student / Former Camrose EMS Manager* / Lifelong EMS Friend / Book 2 "Between Life & Death" Primary Sponsor

  - **Shelly Nolan RN** / *ATLS Coordinator*

- **Tanya Blades EMT-P** / *Past Student / Co-Instructor / Practicum Placements /* Lifelong Friend

- **Tim Essington EMT-P** / *Co-Instructor / Former Manager of EMS Programs / ACP CEO / EMS Co-worker / Partner /* Lifelong Friend

- **Wes Baerg EMT-P** / *Past Student / Co-Instructor / Beaver EMS Manager ITLS Co-Instructor /* Lifelong Friend

GLOSSARY

Completed by many current electronic sources and blended for information purposes only to clarify common terms from (MERCK Manual, Wikipedia, ACP Website, Medscape, http://emedicine.medscape.com/specialties and https://medlineplus.gov/)

Adrenalin - is a hormone, neurotransmitter and medication. Epinephrine is normally produced by both the adrenal glands and certain neurons. It plays an important role in the fight-or-flight response by increasing blood flow to muscles, output of the heart, pupil dilation, and blood sugar. (It does this by binding to alpha and beta receptors).

Advocate(s) - We all have a passion or a cause that we care about. Being an advocate for that cause is always the right thing to do. Have your voice heard. Help those who cannot help themselves.

Automated External Defibrillator (AED) - is a portable electronic device that automatically diagnoses the life-threatening cardiac arrhythmias of ventricular fibrillation and pulseless ventricular tachycardia in a patient, and able to treat them through defibrillation, the application of electrical therapy which stops the arrhythmia, allowing the heart to re-establish an effective rhythm.

Alcohol Ignition Interlocking System (AIIS) - is a breathalyzer for an individual's vehicle. It requires the driver to blow into a mouthpiece on the device before starting the vehicle. If the resultant breath-alcohol concentration analyzed result is greater than the programmed blood alcohol concentration (which varies between countries), the device prevents the engine from being started. The interlock device is located inside the vehicle, near the driver's seat, and is directly connected to the engine's ignition system.

Advanced Life Support (ALS) -is a set of life-saving protocols and skills that extend Basic Life Support to further support the circulation and provide an open airway and adequate ventilation (breathing)

Amiodarone - is an antiarrhythmic medication used to treat and prevent many different types of irregular heartbeats. This includes ventricular tachycardia (VT), ventricular fibrillation (VF), and wide complex tachycardia, as well as atrial fibrillation and paroxysmal supraventricular tachycardia. It can be given by mouth, intravenously, or intraosseous.

Anesthesia - is a state of temporary induced loss of sensation or awareness.

Anesthesiologist - is the doctor that uses this medical speciality that focuses on perioperative medicine and the administration of anesthesia.

Angiocath - a hollow flexible tube for insertion into a body cavity, duct, or vessel to allow the passage of fluids or distend a passageway. Its uses include the drainage of urine from the bladder through the urethra or insertion through a blood vessel into the heart for diagnostic purposes.

Arterial Blood Gas (ABG) - is a test of blood from an artery; it is a blood test that measures the amounts of certain gases (such as oxygen and carbon dioxide) dissolved in arterial blood.

Asystole – is the absence of ventricular contractions lasting longer than the minimum possible to sustain life (about 2 seconds for a human).

Audible crackles - are the clicking, rattling, or crackling noises that may be made by one or both lungs of a human with a respiratory disease during inhalation. They are often heard only with a stethoscope ("on auscultation"), and sometimes can be heard without a stethoscope.

Auscultate - to listen, for diagnostic purposes, to the sounds made by the internal organs of the body.

Battle's Sign - also *mastoid ecchymosis*, is an indication of fracture of middle cranial fossa of the skull, and may suggest underlying brain trauma. Battle's sign consists of bruising over the mastoid process, a result of extravasation of blood along the path of the posterior auricular artery.

Blood Pressure (BP) - is the pressure of circulating blood on the walls of blood vessels. When used without further specification, "blood pressure" usually refers to the pressure in large arteries of the systemic circulation. Blood pressure is usually expressed in terms of the systolic pressure (maximum during one heartbeat) over diastolic pressure (minimum in between two heartbeats) and is measured in millimeters of mercury (mmHg), above the surrounding atmospheric pressure (considered to be zero for convenience).

Basic Life Support (BLS) - is a level of medical care which is used for victims of life-threatening illnesses or injuries until they can be given full medical care at a hospital. It can be provided by trained medical personnel, including emergency medical technicians, paramedics, and by qualified bystanders.

Beats per minute (Bpm) - Cardiac pacing, the unit of measure for the frequency of heart depolarizations or contractions each minute–or pulse rate.

Brain Natriuretic Peptide (BNP) - (also *ventricular natriuretic peptide or natriuretic peptide B*) is a 32-amino acid polypeptide secreted by the ventricles of the heart in response to excessive stretching of heart muscle cells (cardiomyocytes). The release of BNP is modulated by calcium ions. BNP is named as such because it was originally identified in extracts of porcine brain, although in humans it is produced mainly in the cardiac ventricles.

Cardiac Arrest - is a sudden stop in effective blood flow due to the failure of the heart to contract effectively. Symptoms include loss of consciousness and abnormal or absent breathing. Some people may have chest pain, shortness of breath, or nausea before this occurs. If not treated within minutes, death usually occurs.

Cardiac contusion – (*myocardial contusion*) is a term for a bruise (contusion) to the heart after an injury. It is usually a consequence of blunt trauma to the anterior chest wall, and the right ventricle is thought to be most commonly affected due to its anatomic location as the most anterior surface of the heart.

Cardiac Disease - *cardiovascular disease* (CVD) is a class of diseases that involve the heart or blood vessels. Cardiovascular disease includes coronary artery diseases (CAD) such as angina and myocardial infarction (commonly known as a heart attack). Other CVDs include stroke, heart failure, hypertensive heart disease, rheumatic heart disease, cardiomyopathy, heart arrhythmia, congenital heart disease, valvular heart disease, carditis, aortic aneurysms, peripheral artery disease, thromboembolic disease, and venous thrombosis.

Cardiac Care Unit (CCU) - a specialized hospital unit that is specially equipped to treat and monitor patients with serious heart conditions.

Cerebral perfusion (CPP) - is the pressure gradient between the systemic blood pressure and the pressure in the cranial compartment. The pressure difference is the gradient that is necessary to "drive" blood from the aorta into the cranial compartment. Blood flow and perfusion to the brain depend upon an adequate blood pressure gradient.

Cervical Collar - also known as a *neck brace*, is a medical device used to support a person's neck. It is also used by emergency personnel for those who have had traumatic head or neck injuries, and can be used to treat chronic medical conditions.

Child Abuse - child maltreatment is physical, sexual, or psychological mistreatment or neglect of a child or children, especially by a parent or other caregiver. It may include any act or failure to act by a parent or other caregiver that results in actual or potential harm to a child, and can occur in a child's home, or in the organizations, schools or communities the child interacts with.

Compassionate Fatigue - also known as secondary traumatic stress (STS), is a condition characterized by a gradual lessening of compassion over time. It is common among individuals that work directly with trauma victims such as, therapists (paid and unpaid), nurses, teachers, psychologists, police officers, paramedics, animal welfare workers, health unit coordinators and anyone who helps others, especially family members, relatives, and other informal caregivers of patients suffering from a chronic illness.

Complication(s) - in medicine, an unanticipated problem that arises following, and is a result of, a procedure, treatment, or illness. A complication is so named because it complicates the situation.

Computer Aided Dispatch (CAD) - is a computer system that assists 911 operators and dispatch personnel in handling and prioritizing calls. Enhanced 911 will send the location of the call to the CAD system that will automatically display the address of the 911 caller on a screen in front of the operator. Complaint information is then entered into the computer and is easily retrievable. The system may be linked to MDTs in patrol cars allowing dispatchers and officers to communicate without using voice. The system may also be interfaced with NCIC, AVL, or number of other programs

Computer Tomography (CT) is a radiography in which a three-dimensional image of a body structure is constructed by computer from a series of plane cross-sectional images made along an axis.

Congestive Heart Failure (CHF) - heart failure in which the heart is unable to maintain adequate circulation of blood in the tissues of the body or to pump out the venous blood returned to it by the venous circulation.

Conscious - is the state or quality of awareness, or, of being aware of an external object or something within oneself.

Consequences - that which follows something on which it depends; that which is produced by a cause. A result of actions, especially if such a result is unwanted or unpleasant.

Cardiopulmonary Resuscitation (CPR) - an emergency procedure in which the heart and lungs are made to work by compressing the chest overlying the heart and forcing air into the lungs. CPR is used to maintain circulation when the heart has stopped pumping on its own.

Cricothyrotomy - is an incision made through the skin and cricothyroid membrane to establish a patent airway during certain life-threatening situations, such as airway obstruction by a foreign body, angioedema, or massive facial trauma. Cricothyrotomy is nearly always performed as a last resort in cases where endotracheal and nasotracheal intubation are impossible or contraindicated.

Critical Incident Stress Debriefing (CISD) - is a specific, 7-phase, small group, supportive crisis intervention process. It is just one of the many crisis intervention techniques which are included under the umbrella of a Critical Incident Stress Management (CISM) program. The CISD is simply a supportive, crisis-focused discussion of a traumatic event (which is frequently called a "critical incident"). The Critical Incident Stress Debriefing was developed exclusively for small, homogeneous groups who have encountered a powerful traumatic event. It aims at reduction of distress and a restoration of group cohesion and unit performance.

Crystal Meth - is a strong central nervous system (CNS) stimulant that is mainly used as a recreational drug. Methamphetamine is often used recreationally for its effects as a potent euphoriant and stimulant as well as aphrodisiac qualities.

Decompensated Shock - this phase occurs when local tissue beds that were vasoconstricted begin to vasodilate. Vasodilation leads to pooling of blood and maldistribution of flow to "non-essential" organs. Clinical signs include grey mucous membranes, bradycardia, loss of vasomotor tone leading to hypotension, and severely altered mentation. The patient is often stuporous to comatose. Ventricular arrhythmias can be seen on an ECG. It is important to realize that the progression from compensated to decompensated shock can occur over minutes to hours depending on the cause and severity of injury, and that patients can present anywhere along this spectrum.

Diaphoretic - the secretion of sweat, especially the profuse secretion associated with an elevated body temperature, physical exertion, exposure to heat, and mental or emotional stress. Sweating is centrally controlled by the sympathetic nervous system and is primarily a thermoregulatory mechanism. However, the sweat glands on the palms and soles respond to emotional stimuli and do not always participate in thermal sweating. The rate of sweating is generally not affected by water deficiency, but it may be reduced by severe dehydration; it also diminishes when salt intake exceeds salt loss.

Distention - the state of being distended, enlarged, swollen from internal pressure.

Dopamine Infusion - is an organic chemical of the catecholamine and phenethylamine families that plays several important roles in the brain and body. Dopamine as a manufactured medication is most commonly used as a stimulant drug in the treatment of severe low blood pressure, slow heart rate, and cardiac arrest. It is given intravenously. Since the half-life of dopamine in plasma is very short—approximately one minute in adults, two minutes in newborn infants and up to five minutes in preterm infants—it is usually given in a continuous intravenous drip rather than a single injection.

Drug induced haze - caused by recreational or medical drugs; something suggesting atmospheric haze and/or vagueness of mind or mental perception.

Drug seeker - *drug-seeking behavior* (DSB); a pattern of seeking narcotic pain medication or tranquilizers with forged prescriptions, false identification, repeated requests for replacement of "lost" drugs or prescriptions, complaints of severe pain without an organic basis, and abusive or threatening behavior manifested when denied drugs.

Emergency Medical Services (EMS) - is a type of emergency service dedicated to providing out-of-hospital acute medical care, transport to definitive care, and other medical transport to patients with illnesses and injuries which prevent the patient from transporting themselves.

Emergency Medicine - a medical specialty concerned with the care and treatment of acutely ill or injured patients who need immediate medical attention.

EMT-A - a health care provider of emergency medical services. EMTs are clinicians, trained to respond quickly to emergency situations regarding medical issues, traumatic injuries and accident scenes.

End Tidal C02 - *End-tidal capnography* (end-tidal CO2, PETCO2, ET CO2) refers to the graphical measurement of carbon dioxide partial pressure (mm Hg) during expiration. With continuous technological advancements, end-tidal carbon dioxide monitoring has become a key component in the advancement of patient safety.

Entonox - *Nitrous oxide*, sold under the brand name Entonox; is an inhaled gas used as a pain medication and together with other medications for anesthesia. Common uses include during childbirth, following trauma, and as part of end of life care. Onset of effect is typically within half a minute and lasts for about a minute.

ePCR – is an electronic method of patient care reporting used by emergency medical trained personnel to report what care was being done each time the EMS is dispatched for any type of response. Provides call details, basic patient information, history and assessment to interventions.

Epinephrine - a hormone produced by the adrenal medulla; called also *adrenaline* (British). Its function is to aid in the regulation of the sympathetic branch of the autonomic nervous system. At times when a person is highly stimulated, as by fear, anger, or some challenging situation, extra amounts of epinephrine are released into the bloodstream, preparing the body for energetic action. Epinephrine is a powerful vasopressor that increases blood pressure and increases the heart rate and cardiac output. It also increases glycogenolysis and the release of glucose from the liver, so that a person has a suddenly increased feeling of muscular strength and aggressiveness.

Extubate - removal of a previously inserted tube, such as an endotracheal tube, catheter, drain, or feeding tube, from an organ, orifice, or other body structure.

Fast Scan - *Focussed Assessment with Sonography for Trauma* (FAST) scan - is a point-of-care ultrasound examination performed at the time of presentation of a trauma patient. It is invariably performed by a clinician, who should be formally trained, and is considered as an 'extension' of the trauma clinical assessment process, to aid rapid decision making.

Fentanyl - is a potent, synthetic opioid pain medication with a rapid onset and short duration of action. It is a potent agonist of μ-opioid receptors in the brain.

First Responder - a person (such as a police officer or an EMT) who is among those responsible for going immediately to the scene of an accident or emergency to provide assistance.

Glasgow Coma Scale (GCS) - is a neurological scale which aims to give a reliable and objective way of recording the conscious state of a person for initial as well as subsequent assessment. A patient is assessed against the criteria of the scale; the scale is composed of three tests: eye, verbal and motor responses. The three values separately as well as their sum are considered. The lowest possible GCS (the sum) is 3 (deep coma or death), while the highest is 15 (fully awake person).

GCS was initially used to assess level of consciousness after head injury, and the scale is now used by first responders, EMS, nurses and doctors as being applicable to all acute medical and trauma patients. At the hospital, it's also used in monitoring chronic patients in intensive care.

Health Professions Act (HPA) - majority of health professions are regulated by self governing colleges under the HPA. All regulated health professions will eventually come under the HPA. The HPA was developed to regulate health professions using a model that allows for non-exclusive, overlapping scopes of practice. No single profession has exclusive ownership of a specific skill or health service and different professions may provide the same health services.

Health Worker - are all the people who are engaged in actions whose primary intent is to enhance health.

Hemoglobin (Hgb) - the red coloring matter of the red blood corpuscles, a protein yielding heme and globin on hydrolysis: it carries oxygen from the lungs to the tissues, and carbon dioxide from the tissues to the lungs.

Hemothorax - is a type of pleural effusion in which blood accumulates in the pleural cavity. This excess fluid can interfere with normal breathing by limiting the expansion of the lungs.

Human Evolution - is the evolutionary process that led to the emergence of anatomically modern humans.

Hyperventilating - (also called *over-breathing*) occurs when the rate and quantity of alveolar ventilation of carbon dioxide exceeds the body's production of carbon dioxide.

Hypovolemic - is a state of decreased blood volume; more specifically, decrease in volume of blood plasma. It is thus the intravascular component of volume contraction (or loss of blood volume due to things such as bleeding or dehydration), but, as it also is the most essential one.

Hypoxic heart - is a condition in which the body or a region of the body is deprived of adequate oxygen supply at the tissue level, in this case it involves the heart.

Intervention(s) - the act of intervening, interfering or interceding with the intent of modifying the outcome. In medicine, an intervention is usually undertaken to help treat or cure a condition.

Interventional Cardiac Catheter Lab – a specialized area where a cardiac catheterization (heart catheterization) procedure is performed. It's the insertion of a catheter into a chamber or vessel of the heart. This is done both for diagnostic and interventional purposes. Subsets of this technique are mainly coronary catheterization, involving the catheterization of the coronary arteries, and catheterization of cardiac chambers and valves of the cardiac system.

Interventional Radiology Procedures - interventional radiologists (IRs) use their expertise in reading X-rays, ultrasound and other medical images to guide small instruments such as catheters (tubes that measure just a few millimeters in diameter) through the blood vessels or other pathways to treat disease percutaneously (through the skin). These procedures are typically much less invasive and much less costly than traditional surgery.

Intraosseous - is the process of injecting directly into the marrow of a bone to provide a non-collapsible entry point into the systemic venous system. This technique is used to provide fluids and medication when intravenous access is not available or not feasible.

International Trauma Life Support (ITLS) - is a global not-for-profit organization dedicated to preventing death and disability from trauma through education and emergency trauma care. ITLS courses give the student the knowledge and hands-on skills to take better care of trauma patients. ITLS stresses rapid assessment, appropriate intervention and identification of immediate life threats. The ITLS framework for rapid, appropriate and effective trauma care is a global standard that works in any situation.

Jaws of Life - emergency rescue equipment used to open a destroyed passenger vehicle, to quickly and somewhat safely extricate the trapped occupants.

Laryngoscope - a rigid or flexible endoscope passed through the mouth and equipped with a source of light and magnification, for examining and performing local diagnostic and surgical procedures on the larynx.

Left main coronary artery (LMCA) - is one of the coronary arteries that arises from the aorta above the left cusp of the aortic valve and feeds blood to the left side of the heart.

Level of consciousness (LOC) - is a measurement of a person's arousability and responsiveness to stimuli from the environment.

Levophed - *norepinephrine bitartrate* is an adjunctive treatment in cardiac arrest and profound hypotension. Levophed functions as a peripheral vasoconstrictor (alpha-adrenergic action) and as an inotropic stimulator of the heart and dilator of coronary arteries (beta-adrenergic action).

Life threatening – when there is an illness or situation that there is a strong possibility that it will kill them.

Mannitol - is a naturally occurring substance that causes the body to lose water (diuresis) through osmosis.

Mean Arterial Pressure (MAP) - is a term used in medicine to describe an average blood pressure in an individual. It is defined as the average arterial pressure during a single cardiac cycle.

Medevac - is the timely and efficient movement and en route care provided by medical personnel to wounded being evacuated from a battlefield, to injured patients being evacuated from the scene of an accident to receiving medical facilities, or to patients at a rural hospital requiring urgent care at a better-equipped facility using medically equipped ground vehicles (ambulances) or aircraft (air ambulances).

Medical - relating to the science of medicine, or to the treatment of illness and injuries.

Medication administration - the applying, dispensing, or giving of drugs or medicines as prescribed by a physician.

Mental Health Act - is the law which sets out when you can be admitted, detained and treated in hospital against your wishes.

Mentor- is a person who enters a relationship in which a more experienced or more knowledgeable person helps to guide a less experienced or less knowledgeable person. The mentor may be older or younger than the person being mentored, but he or she must have a certain area of expertise. It is a learning and development partnership between someone with vast experience and someone who wants to learn.

Milliamperes - a unit of electric current that is one thousandth of an ampere. Ampere is the current that, if maintained in two straight parallel conductors of infinite length and of negligible circular cross-sections and placed 1 m apart in a vacuum, produces between them a force of $2 \times 10\text{-}7$ N/m of length.

Mindful Meditation - Mindfulness is the practice of cultivating non-judgemental awareness in day-to-day life. Meditation is a tool, a type of training to help us be more mindful during each day. Benefits people who experience stress in their lives as well as those who don't. It enables us to live our life more fully, effectively, and peacefully. It gives us greater control of our experiences and more satisfying ways of responding to them. It helps us transcend any images of our self and our capabilities that might narrow our experience.

Narcan Kits - is a drug that can be injected to temporarily reverse an overdose of fentanyl or other opioids, allowing the patient to then get emergency medical help. Each kit contains two units of naloxone, two syringes, two alcohol swabs, two latex gloves, a one-way breathing mask and instructions.

Neglect - is a form of abuse where the perpetrator is responsible for caring for someone, who is unable to care for themselves, but fails to do so. Neglect may include the failure to provide sufficient supervision, nourishment, or medical care, or the failure to fulfill other needs for which the victim cannot provide themselves.

Netcare - The EHR is not a single database, but rather a network of data repositories and information systems. Each has an important function and together they form the provincial EHR. Clinical data is collected through point-of-service systems (in hospitals, laboratories, testing facilities, pharmacies, and clinics), and is sent through secure messaging to the provincial repositories and information systems. When a health professional logs on to the EHR through the Alberta Netcare Portal, and searches for a patient record, the portal retrieves all the available information from the provincial systems and presents it as a unified patient record.

Neurogenic Shock - is a distributive type of shock resulting in low blood pressure, occasionally with a slowed heart rate, that is attributed to the disruption of the autonomic pathways within the spinal cord. It can occur after damage to the central nervous system such as spinal cord injury.

Neutralized - render (something) ineffective or harmless by applying an opposite force or effect.

Nitro infusion - *nitroglycerin infusion* is used to treat hypertension (high blood pressure) during surgery or to control congestive heart failure in patients who have had a heart attack. It may also be used to produce hypotension (low blood pressure) during surgery. Nitroglycerin infusion is sometimes used to treat angina (chest pain) in patients who have been treated with other medicines that did not work well.

NRB face mask (NRB) - *a non-rebreather mask* is a device used in medicine to assist in the delivery of oxygen therapy. An NRB requires that the patient can breathe unassisted, but unlike low flow nasal cannula, the NRB allows for the delivery of higher concentrations of oxygen.

On-line medical control – (OLMC) is utilized to provide the prehospital provider medical oversight in the treatment decisions involving patient care in the prehospital setting.

Pediatric Advanced Life Support (PALS) - is a video-based, Instructor-led, advanced course, that focuses on a systematic approach to pediatric assessment, basic life support, PALS treatment algorithms, effective resuscitation and team dynamics to improve the quality of care provided to seriously ill or injured children, resulting in improved outcomes.

Pan Scan - whole-body CT scans can confirm immediately whether severe trauma patients have certain injuries, but these tests could miss other serious problems if performed too early. It has been found that single-pass whole-body [CT] is very effective or specific at determining where there is injured tissue but is variable in excluding injuries in patients with suspected blunt trauma.

Paramedic – EMT-P / PCP / ACP or CCP is a healthcare professional, predominantly in the pre-hospital and out-of-hospital environment, and working mainly as part of emergency medical services (EMS), such as on an ambulance.

Perfectionist - is a personality trait characterized by a person's striving for flawlessness and setting high performance standards, accompanied by critical self-evaluations and concerns regarding others' evaluations. It is best conceptualized as a multidimensional characteristic, as psychologists agree that there are many positive and negative aspects.

Personal Protective Equipment (PPE) - refers to protective clothing, helmets, goggles, or other garments or equipment designed to protect the wearer's body from injury or infection. The hazards addressed by protective equipment include physical, electrical, heat, chemicals, biohazards, and airborne particulate matter.

Pharmacology - is the branch of biology concerned with the study of drug action, where a drug can be broadly defined as any man-made, natural, or endogenous (from within body) molecule which exerts a biochemical or physiological effect on the cell, tissue, organ, or organism.

Pleural Effusion - is a buildup of fluid in the pleural space, an area between the layers of tissue that line the lungs and the chest cavity. This excess can impair breathing by limiting the expansion of the lungs. Various kinds of pleural effusion, depending on the nature of the fluid and what caused its entry into the pleural space.

Pleural Tap – is a procedure which involves the removal of fluid from the area between the chest cavity and the tissue lining of the lungs.

Pneumonia - is an inflammatory condition of the lung affecting primarily the microscopic air sacs known as alveoli.

Practitioner(s) - a person actively engaged in an art, discipline, or profession, especially medicine.

Preceptor - a preceptor is a skilled practitioner or faculty member who supervises students in a clinical setting to allow practical experience with patients.

Pressor - an antihypotensive agent, also known as a *vasopressor agent*, is any medication that tends to raise reduced blood pressure. Some antihypotensive drugs act as vasoconstrictors to increase total peripheral resistance, others sensitize adrenoreceptors to catecholamines-glucocorticoids, and the third class increase cardiac output-dopamine, such as dobutamine.

Primary Care Paramedic (PCPs) - are the entry-level of para-medic practice in some Canadian provinces. The scope of practice includes performing semi-automated external defibrillation. Oxygen administration. Establishing an IV. Cardiac monitoring such as Lead 2 and 12 Lead interpretation. Administration of Symptom Relief Medications for a variety of emergency medical conditions (these include epinephrine, salbutamol, ipratropium bromide, aspirin, nitroglycerine, naloxone, dextrose, thiamine, glucagon, gravol, benadryl and nitrous oxide). In addition, some services have started implementing non-opiate medications so that Primary Care Paramedics can treat patients that require pain management. These medications include ketorolac, acetaminophen and ibuprofen. As of 2015, PCP's can now administer Naloxone for suspected opiate overdose. Performing trauma immobilization, including cervical immobilization, and other basic medical care. PCPs may also receive additional training to perform certain skills that are normally in the scope of practice of ACPs, such as interpretation or transmission of a 12 lead EKG. This is regulated both provincially (by statute) and locally (by the medical director), and ordinarily entails an aspect of medical oversight by a specific body or group of physicians. See https://www.collegeofparamedics.org/ for more information.

Priority One - the emergency services in various countries use systems of response codes to categorize their responses to reported events. To describe a mode of response for an emergency vehicle responding to a call. Some Paramedic/EMS agencies use Priority terms, which run in the opposite of code responses.

> Priority 1 - Dead On Arrival Trauma/CPR
> Priority 2 - Emergency
> Priority 3 - Non- Emergency
> Priority 4 - Situation Under Control
> Priority 5 - Mass Casualty

Post Traumatic Stress Disorder (PTSD) - is a disorder that develops in some people who have experienced a shocking, scary, or dangerous event. Not everyone with PTSD has been through a dangerous event. Some experiences, like the sudden, unexpected death of a loved one, can also cause PTSD. Symptoms usually begin early, within 3 months of the traumatic incident, but sometimes they begin years afterward. Symptoms must last more than a month and be severe enough to interfere with relationships or work to be considered PTSD.

Rapid Sequence Intubation (RSI) - is a special process for endotracheal intubation that is used where the patient is at a high risk of pulmonary aspiration or impending airway compromise. It differs from other forms of general anesthesia induction in that artificial ventilation is generally not provided from the time the patient stops breathing (when drugs are given) until after intubation has been achieved.

Royal Canadian Mounted Police (RCMP) - is both a federal and a national police force of Canada. The RCMP provides law enforcement at a federal level in Canada, also on a contract basis to the three territories, eight of Canada's provinces (the RCMP does not provide provincial or municipal policing in either Ontario or Quebec), more than 150 municipalities, 600 aboriginal communities, and three international airports. http://www.rcmp.gc.ca/

Sellick's Maneuver - *cricoid pressure*, is a technique used in endotracheal intubation to reduce the risk of regurgitation. The technique involves the application of pressure to the cricoid cartilage at the neck, thus occluding the esophagus which passes directly behind it. (Only to be done by specially trained providers)

Sinus Bradycardia - is a heart rhythm that originates in the sinus node with a rates less than 60 beats per minute. Common in healthy patients but not in sick patients who are hypoxic, hypovolemic or something that is causing the bradycardia.

ST Segment monitoring - is useful for detecting silent ischemia. ST-segment monitoring is more sensitive than patients self-reporting of symptoms because 70% to 90% of episodes of myocardial ischemia detected with ECG are clinically silent.

Standard of Care - is the watchfulness, attention, caution and prudence that a reasonable person in the circumstances would exercise.

STARS – (Shock Trauma Air Rescue Society) is a dedicated flight team that provides safe, rapid, highly specialized emergency medical transport system for the critically ill and injured. It offers time, hope and life-saving transport. Currently in Alberta, Saskatchewan, and Manitoba although the odd flight does extend into BC for the Calgary Flight Crews from time to time. See https://www.stars.ca/

Stroke disease - stroke is a disease that affects the arteries leading to and within the brain. It is the No. 5 cause of death and a leading cause of disability in the United States. A stroke occurs when a blood vessel that carries oxygen and nutrients to the brain is either blocked by a clot or bursts (or ruptures).

Subconscious - is the part of consciousness that is not currently in focal awareness.

Subcutaneous Emphysema - is when gas or air is in the layer under the skin. Subcutaneous refers to the tissue beneath the skin, and emphysema refers to trapped air.

Surgical - is an ancient medical specialty that uses operative manual and instrumental techniques on a patient to investigate or treat a pathological condition such as disease or injury, to help improve bodily function or appearance or to repair unwanted ruptured areas.

Surreal - marked by the intense irrational reality of a dream; unbelievable, fantastic.

Tactical Officer - specially trained officers to deal with certain high-risk situations, dealing with some of the most complex and dangerous situations.

Technological - technology can be the knowledge of techniques, processes, and the like, or it can be embedded in machines which can be operated without detailed knowledge of their workings.

Therapeutic Touch - is a natural healing method for relaxation and self-help. It relieves pain, stress and anxiety, improves sleep and well-being.

Third Degree Heart Block - is a disorder of the cardiac conduction system where there is no conduction through the atrioventricular node (AVN). Therefore, complete dissociation of the atrial and ventricular activity exists. The ventricular escape mechanism can occur anywhere from the AVN to the bundle-branch Purkinje system.

Tragedies - an event causing great suffering, destruction, and distress, such as a serious accident, crime, or natural catastrophe.

Tranexamic Acid – (TXA) is a synthetic analog of the amino acid lysine. It is used to treat or prevent excessive blood loss during surgery and in various medical conditions or disorders (helping hemostasis).

Traumatic - emotionally disturbing or distressing. We commonly use along with any trauma or with the term a traumatic event that includes many issues. it when something is broken due to force, displaced parts, falling apart due to excessive force, injury from force or is from an unnatural event commonly.

Traumatic Event - is an experience that causes physical, emotional, psychological distress, or harm. It is an event that is perceived and experienced as a threat to one's safety or to the stability of one's world.

Type 2 Acute Myocardial Infarction (Type 2 MI)– is the early critical stage of necrosis of heart muscle tissue caused by blockage of a coronary artery. It is characterized by elevated S-T segments in the reflecting leads and elevated levels of cardiac enzymes. Type 2 myocardial infarction mortality was concluded to be more likely due to the nature of the myocardial infarction rather than comorbidities, and independent of the underlying triggering conditions that led to it.

Type 2 Atrioventricular Block (Type 2 Second-degree AV block) - also known as "Mobitz II," is almost always a disease of the distal conduction system (His-Purkinje System). Mobitz II heart block is characterized on a surface ECG by intermittently non-conducted P waves not preceded by PR prolongation and not followed by PR shortening.

Unconscious – insensible; incapable of responding to sensory stimuli and of having subjective experiences. (GCS 3/15)

Ventolin - a beta-agonist bronchodilator that is administered in the form of its sulfate, as an inhalational aerosol or as a tablet to treat bronchospasm associated especially with asthma and chronic obstructive pulmonary disease.

Dale M. Bayliss

Ventricular Fibrillation (V Fib) - an often, fatal heartbeat irregularity in which the muscle fibers of the ventricles work without coordination and cause a loss of effective pumping action of the heart.

Ventricular Tachycardia (V-tach) - is a rapid heartbeat that originates in one of the lower chambers (the ventricles) of the heart. To be classified as tachycardia, the heart rate is usually at least 100 beats per minute.

CPSIA information can be obtained
at www.ICGtesting.com
Printed in the USA
LVOW08s1755180118
563129LV00009B/601/P